Dental Nursing
NVQ III

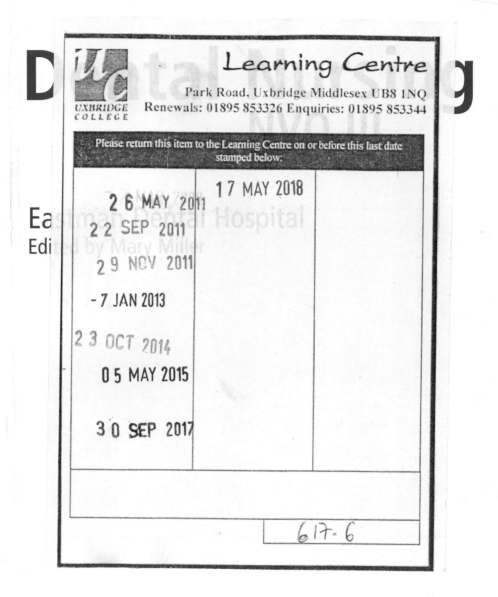

Eastman Dental Hospital
Edited by Mary Miller

Hodder Arnold
A MEMBER OF THE HODDER HEADLINE GROUP

Orders: please contact Bookpoint Ltd, 130 Milton Park, Abingdon, Oxon OX14 4SB. Telephone: (44) 01235 827720. Fax: (44) 01235 400454. Lines are open from 9.00–6.00, Monday to Saturday, with a 24 hour message answering service. You can also order through our website www.hoddereducation.co.uk

British Library Cataloguing in Publication Data
A catalogue record for this title is available from the British Library

ISBN-10: 0 340 813008
ISBN-13: 978 340 81300 3

First Published 2003

Impression number   10 9 8 7 6 5 4 3 2
Year   2007 2006 2005

Cover photo from James King-Holmes/Science Photo Library
Typeset by Pantek Arts Ltd, Maidstone, Kent.
Printed in Great Britain for Hodder Education, a division of Hodder Headline Plc, 338 Euston Road, London NW1 3BH by Martins The Printers Ltd

CONTENTS

LIST OF AUTHORS

Chapter 1 Communication: Jay Daniels

Chapter 2 Equality, diversity and rights: Jacqueline Jackson

Chapter 3 Medical Emergencies: Wendy Irving

Chapter 4 Cross Infection Control: Angela Luke, Mary Miller, and Julie Rolink

Chapter 5 Dental Radiography: Fiona Ball

Chapter 6 Oral Health and the Prevention of Periodontal Disease and Dental Caries: Jay Daniels

Chapter 7 Conservation: Jane Sims

Chapter 8 Dental Implants: Amanda Best

Chapter 9 Paediatric Dentistry: Mary Miller and Helen Richardson

Chapter 10 Orthodontics: Jay Daniels

Chapter 11 Minor Oral Surgery: Mary Miller

Chapter 12 Prosthetics: Wendy Irving

Chapter 13 Conscious Sedation: Helen Richardson

ACKNOWLEDGEMENTS

This book is dedicated to David Rule 17th April 1937 – 29th August 2000 for his support and encouragement in the training and education of dental nurses.

The author team would like to express their gratitude to Mr Victor Crow, Consultant Orthodontist, Hillingdon Hospital, and Central Middlesex Hospital; also to Dr Henry Schofield, Alan Stoltz, John Richards, Corrine Willson, and Christopher Edwards.

INTRODUCTION

The care of patients receiving dental treatment is of paramount importance to everyone involved in dentistry. All members of the dental team have a vital role to play and it is essential that all receive the correct training and education.

This book has (in the main) been written by dental nurses for dental nurses in light of statutory registration and is intended to meet a need for information and guidance in conjunction with the training dental nurses receive during courses or working day-to-day in a practice. It is intended not only as an information source for unqualified dental nurses, but also as an aide memoire for qualified dental nurses.

The chapters are all linked to the NVQ Level 3 in Oral Health Care – Dental Nursing and are fully illustrated with diagrams, photos and charts. The subject matters covered in each chapter are not intended to be exhaustive, but reflect the units that are required for qualification.

During the text, you will see some symbols. A 'pointing finger' ☞ indicates that the passage is of special significance and particularly relates to the role of the dental nurse.

Of course there are lots of other sources of information for the dental nurse. Ask lots of questions and get the dental team to question you; learn the names of instruments, burs and other items used within a practice; read the instructions on dental materials; the list of what you can do is endless and remember …

'if you really want to do something you will find a way. If you do not you will find an excuse'.

COMMUNICATION
Linked to DN17

Introduction

This chapter is linked to DN17 of the NVQ Level 3 in Oral Health Care.

Good communication is an important and vital skill for all health professionals to possess. The dental nurse (DN) is no exception, being a vital link between the patient and the dentist. They are often required to pass on information about treatment and give oral health education.

There is the old saying, 'It's not *what* you say but the *way* you say it'. The way a person looks, their body language, tone and level of voice can all have an influence on the way a person responds to what is being said to them. Communication is a complex process, which involves many variables including environment, age, social class, language, gender, culture, religion and experience.

One of the main reasons for communicating is to exchange information. Access to appropriate, high quality information empowers an individual to make certain decisions, enabling them to change their lifestyle and improve their health and, ultimately, their quality of life. In the dental environment, information is generally received or passed on through direct person-to-person interaction, and therefore an important aspect of communication is to be able to quickly establish positive relationships with the many different types of people you will be in contact with throughout the working day. When we look at communication, we cannot divorce it from the context in which it occurs and the people it involves.

This chapter will cover:

○ Communication breakdown

○ Communication techniques including verbal and non-verbal

○ Other factors that affect communication

○ Dealing with anxiety in the dental surgery through communication

SECTION 1: Communication breakdown

When communication breaks down trust and respect can be lost. Since no one is infallible, it is inevitable that some communication failures and problems will occur.

Information overload

When people are given too much information, the result may be a kind of paralysis, caused by an inability to see the wood for the trees. They have to spend most of their time sifting through all the information given trying to sort out what is important from a mass of unnecessary information.

Insufficient information

Too little information can also lead to inactivity because no one has the necessary information to progress with confidence. Individuals may put their own interpretation on the messages being received resulting in inappropriate or incorrect oral health care.

Ineffective communication

Communication that doesn't lead to the desired outcome may be well intentioned, but it may be misplaced, inaccurate or incomplete.

SECTION 2: Communication techniques

Verbal communication

Complex speech is unique to human beings. Other animals do use forms of communication that may constitute a language; however, we have yet to discover a language system as diverse and complex as our own. Speech is the most common form of communication, and as such we tend to take it for granted. There are many factors that can affect verbal communication either to enhance it or hinder it (Table 1).

Positive	Negative
Appropriate level of tone	Shouting/whispering
Speaking in a clear voice	Mumbling
Speaking at a steady and appropriate pace	Speaking too quickly or too slowly
Facing the person you are speaking to	Looking down or away from the person to whom you are speaking
Uncovered mouth	Mouth covered with a hand or mask (for example)
Clean teeth	Plaque covered, stained teeth
Sweet breath	Halitosis (alcohol, garlic)
Allowing time for response	Not allowing time for a response
Interrupting the other person only when absolutely necessary	Always interrupting the other person
Not finishing off the other person's sentences	Constantly finishing off the other person's sentences

Table 1: Factors that can affect communication

Non-verbal communication

Non-verbal communication can be either positive or negative, i.e. complement or work against verbal communication (Table 2). Such things as body language, eye contact and hand gestures can communicate to another person what you are really feeling, and whether your words are as sincere and truthful as they may sound.

Some negative non-verbal communication may be just a bad habit that needs modifying, or it may be used intentionally to intimidate or show a lack of interest to the other person. Positive non-verbal communication can be used very effectively with people who have learning disabilities, do not have English as a first language or who have a hearing impairment. It can also work well with young children and nervous patients (simply smile!).

Positive	Negative
Appropriate eye contact (but not for long periods)	Looking anywhere but at the person – especially at your watch or at the clock behind the person's head
Body in a relaxed 'open' pose	A rigid body pose with folded arms, or a far too relaxed body pose that may be interpreted in an over friendly or sexual way. Fidgeting
Try and position yourself at the same height to the person you are speaking to	Standing above the person or sitting behind a desk and making them stand
Keeping an appropriate amount of distance or personal space between you and the person you are communicating with	Encroaching on an individual's 'personal' space, or positioning yourself at a great distance
An interested expression	A bored expression accompanied by yawning. If you really have to yawn, cover your mouth and apologise
Smile occasionally	Never smile
Occasional nodding with head slightly to one side	Rigid, upright head, with no nodding
Not eating or chewing gum	Eating and chewing gum
Total attention to person	Having conversations with other people. Allowing interruptions

Table 2: Non-verbal communications

SECTION 3: Other factors that affect communication

As mentioned in the introduction to this chapter, there are many factors that affect communication. These may include environment, language, disabilities, gender, culture and religion.

Environment

A busy dental surgery can often be a noisy bustling place, which may lead to communication difficulties, especially with nervous or upset patients. Try to create and maintain a quiet and relaxed atmosphere both in the reception and clinical area. Reduce noise levels by closing windows/doors, turning off radios and not shouting across to colleagues or calling to other patients from a distance. If you are finding it difficult to have a conversation with a patient due to disruption or noise levels, try and take them to another room or an area that may be quieter.

A patient may be distracted by an untidy or dirty environment, or feel that professional standards are not being adhered to, leading to communication breakdown. Try to keep the reception and clinical environment clean, tidy and free from clutter. Put unnecessary items away and try not to have lots of notes or empty boxes lying around. Make sure bins are not overflowing and the reading material in the waiting area is periodically tidied. By adhering to health and safety regulations and infection control procedures, the clinical environment will automatically stay safe, clean and tidy.

Attempt to reduce or minimise interruptions when treating a patient or talking to them about personal dental health matters. Put on the answer-phone, put a 'do not disturb' sign on the door or ask other members of staff not to disturb you whilst with a patient. Try and maintain a constant comfortable room temperature (21°C), and reduce the possibility of the room becoming too hot, cold or draughty.

Language

Some patients or visitors to the dental practice may not have English as a first language and this will inevitably cause some communication difficulties. To enhance effective communication, speak slowly and clearly using positive, non-verbal, communication. If possible, ask the person to bring along an interpreter, such as another family member or friend. Do be aware that in some circumstances it may be a young child who has the responsibility of translating for a parent or another family member, and this can cause difficulties with communicating complex information. It would be better to arrange for an adult to act as interpreter or contact your local NHS Trust who may have an appropriate interpreting service. All professional interpreters follow a code of conduct, which accompanies the National Register of Public Service Interpreters. If the practice does see patients who do not have English as a first language, then information leaflets could be provided in other languages. It may be useful to contact your local oral health promotion unit, which may have leaflets and posters in other languages.

Sensory impairment and physical disabilities

Some patients may have a sensory impairment that affects sight and hearing, and/or physical disabilities. The use of basic sign language, positive non-verbal communication and leaflets in Braille will all contribute to improving communication. Work with the patient and ask them in what ways you can improve communication within the dental environment to suit their needs. Always address the patient directly and never 'talk down to them', as this can be insulting and upsetting. Try and create an environment that is suited to patients in wheelchairs, such as surgeries on the ground floor and disabled toilets with low sinks and mirrors. However, modifying environmental factors to enhance effective communication may be difficult if the dental practice is small and located on upper floors.

Try and provide oral hygiene aids that have been adapted for patients with manual dexterity difficulties, and be prepared to demonstrate their use.

For patients with learning or mental disabilities it may take a little longer to establish a relationship where effective communication is achieved. Ask the person who may be accompanying them, family, key workers or teachers, how best to communicate to suit individual needs.

Visual disability

- Appropriate gentle touching and tone of voice are important
- Speak to the visually impaired person not the accompanying person
- Do not grab them and lead them into the surgery, let them rest their hand on your arm
- Try and provide Braille information leaflets
- Contact the Royal Society for the visually impaired to get information
- Allow them to touch and use all recommended oral hygiene aids
- An electric toothbrush may be helpful
- Do not shout at them
- Always inform them of what procedures are about to take place
- Do not suddenly come up behind them

Hearing disability

- Always look at the person
- Speak slowly, form words carefully and do not mumble
- There is no need to shout
- Provide pen and paper if necessary
- Avoid high pitched background noise when talking as it can affect hearing aids
- It may be useful to learn basic sign language
- Use a gentle touch on the shoulder when you want to attract the patient's attention if they are turned away from you
- Do not suddenly come up behind them
- They may have a side which has better hearing, remember this if the patient informs you

Gender

A person's gender means more than just their physical appearance (e.g. a person's sex); it also includes the social and psychological differences between males and females. Men and women may feel ill at ease in or intimidated by an environment that is predominantly of the opposite gender to themselves, and therefore effective communication will be hindered. The DN should be aware of these potential difficulties and be prepared to accommodate a person if they want to discuss personal matters with someone only of the same gender.

Culture

A person's culture may be described as the way they would normally behave within the society to which they belong. It can be about their value system and what they consider as acceptable behaviour within certain situations. A person's culture can have an effect on communication if the rules of the society in which they live are broken. This could include shouting, impinging on a person's personal space, excessive gesticulation or directing questions only to one person whilst ignoring another. It may be difficult to adapt quickly to other cultural norms when dealing with an upset or nervous patient, and acquiring good communication skills in this situation may only be achieved though experience. However, the majority of cultures would recognise professional behaviour, and therefore this would be a good foundation on which to base effective communication.

Religion

A person's religious beliefs are extremely important to them, and if they feel that they are being ignored or treated differently because of them it will lead to communication breakdown. Although the DN is not expected to know all the different practices of every religion, they should be prepared to understand and try if possible to accommodate a person so that they can adhere to their religious beliefs when attending a dental surgery.

SECTION 4: Dealing with anxiety in the dental environment through effective communication

Many people are anxious about going to the dentist, but it may be too simplistic to assume that it is just the fear of pain that makes them anxious, as many people still will not go even if they are suffering from excruciating toothache. There are many factors that prevent people from attending the dentist, including:

○ Pain

○ The unknown

○ The injection

○ Sounds and tastes

○ Being told off or being given bad news

○ Lying supine

○ Gagging and water in the mouth

○ Catching a disease

Other reasons why people do not attend the dentist regularly may include:

○ Financial implications

○ Time consuming/waiting

○ Not being pleased with results

○ Lack of motivation

○ Embarrassment

○ Too busy

○ Disabled – mentally and physically

○ Age

○ Dirty reception area or surgery

○ Equipment breaking down

○ Lost notes

○ Rude, or untidy staff

There are often simple steps that can be taken to help relieve general patient anxiety when they visit your dental surgery or clinic. These actions are all in some way or another connected with the many factors of communication that have been previously covered in this chapter. Minimise the waiting time for the patient and try and create a pleasant friendly dental environment. Have interesting visual distractions such as up-to-date magazines in good condition or videos. Keep to the appointment time if possible (or have delays explained to your patient).

Introduce yourself to the patient if it is the first time you have met, and use your patient's name more than once during the treatment (check what they like to be called).

Ask the patient about themselves (e.g. what have they been doing, children, holidays etc.), and try to avoid talking about yourself too much or talking to a colleague on personal or social issues whilst ignoring the patient. Show the patient you are listening/understanding by verbal and positive non-verbal communication.

Allow enough time for the patient to get comfortable in the chair before putting it back, tying on bibs, putting on glasses and turning on lights.

Reassure honestly, use touch appropriately and do not 'make up' answers. If you do not know how to respond to the patient's question, ask someone who is in a position to know the answer.

Keep the patient informed on how systems operate in the surgery or clinic (appointments, payments, opening hours, emergency services etc.).

Most importantly, however busy or stressed you feel, do not take it out on the patient, or other colleagues in the presence of a patient. Also, remember to smile, it can reassure a patient and make you feel better!

References
Sociology, Giddens A. 1993 (2nd Ed), Polity Press, Cambridge.

2 EQUALITY, DIVERSITY AND RIGHTS
Linked to DN16

This chapter is linked to the DN16 of the NVQ Level 3 in Oral Health Care, it is also linked to the National Certificate for Dental Nurses Curriculum and will form part of the Continuing Professional Development (CPD) for all members of the dental team.

The chapter will make references throughout to NVQ, but this should not detract from the main message. This chapter will assist the reader to:

❍ Promote the values of equality, diversity and anti-discriminatory practice

❍ Maintain the confidentiality of information

❍ Develop and maintain effective working relationships and appropriate role boundaries

❍ Balance individual rights and choice with the services that the agency delivers

❍ Work within statutory and organisational frameworks

❍ Communicate effectively

Areas that will be covered:

*Promotes people's rights and responsibilities (DN16.1) ☞

KEY WORDS

Context – recognise people's right to make their own decisions in the context of their lives, both socio-economic and personal.

Information – provide up-to-date information in written and unwritten forms (speech, sign, symbols).

Appropriate help – acting on behalf of the person when they are not able to do so/seeking someone else to act on their behalf (interpreter/advocate).

Tensions – within people; between people; between people and agencies.

Appropriate support towards resolution – direct challenges to the people concerned, seek help from others, seek to change the structure and systems that effect people's rights.

*Promote equality and diversity of people (DN16.2) ☞

KEY WORDS

Diversity – individual and social characteristics (age, gender, sexuality, race, health status, relationship status, abilities). Values and beliefs (creed, culture, political beliefs, religion).

Professional frameworks – the worker's actions to promote anti-discriminatory practice.

Appropriate action – to minimise the impact of discrimination/oppression on people (challenge the source of the discrimination and oppression, seek the support of others, seek appropriate support for the person who is being oppressed or discriminated against).

Appropriate support – advice, guidance, counselling, support for the worker/person being oppressed or discriminated against.

*Promote people's rights to the confidentiality of information (DN16.3) ☞

KEY WORDS

Store information – electronically and in writing.

Appropriate precautions – in relation to who might overhear or oversee the information and who might access the information.

Communicating – confidential or sensitive information, electronically, in writing or orally (speech, signing, symbols).

Support – advice from colleagues and others on the action the worker should take, support from colleagues and others to take joint action.

Sharing information – might include information that indicates that the person who told the worker is at risk, that others may be at risk, or indicators of abuse.

SECTION 1:   Religions and beliefs

Since the beginning of recorded time, people with diverse histories, cultures, beliefs and languages have settled in the United Kingdom. Some, like the Huguenots (Protestant refugees who arrived in the 17th century), gradually became assimilated. Others, such as the Irish and Jews, who came at various periods, often maintained separate group identities. People from South Asia, Africa and the Caribbean arrived in substantial numbers after the Second World War to help meet severe labour shortages. The most recent arrivals include refugees and asylum seekers from Vietnam, Somalia, Turkey, the Middle East and former Yugoslavia. Many other people from around the world come to the United Kingdom as workers, students or tourists. The United Kingdom is also home to diverse groups such as people with disabilities and members of the lesbian, gay, bisexual and transgender communities. (Linked to DN16.2)

Buddism

Today, Buddhism is divided into two major branches:

○ *Theravada* has its roots in Sri Lanka and South-east Asia;

○ *Mahayana* has its greatest impact in China, Japan, Tibet, Nepal, Mongolia, Korea, Taiwan, Bhutan and India.

Worship

Buddhists worship in temples or smaller meeting houses (*viharas*). Often, there will be accommodation for Buddhist teachers attached to the temple or vihara. These Buddhist teachers should be addressed as 'Venerable' or 'Sir'.

A shrine can be found in most Buddhist homes. This usually consists of a small table with a statue or image of Buddha surrounded by flowers, candles and sweet smelling incense. When entering a shrine room in a temple or home, headgear and shoes should be removed

Diet

○ Because Buddhism encourages its followers to avoid exploiting living beings, most Buddhists are vegetarians or abstain from eating meat when possible.

○ Humanist (*Mahayana*) Buddhists are extremely strict about their diet and will not eat meat, fish, seafood or gelatine products. There are also five vegetables they will not eat because their odour is believed to attract evil. These vegetables are garlic, onion, leek, spring onion and chives.

○ Monks, nuns and some lay Buddhists may have only one meal a day (at lunchtime).

Dress code

○ Buddhists usually wear the predominant style of dress of the country in which they live.

○ Many Buddhists will wear a necklace or chain with a Buddhist image or icon on it and chanting beads around their wrists. A sensitive approach should be taken if an individual is asked to remove any of these items.

○ Monks and nuns wear different colour robes depending on the country of origin of the monastic tradition in which they take their monastic vows.

○ Monks and nuns wear their hair very short, and in many cases shave their heads.

QUESTIONS

Question 1

a. What 2 branches is Buddhism divided into?

○

○

b. What 5 vegetables are not eaten by Buddhists?

○   ○

○   ○

○

Christianity

About a third of the world's population identify themselves as Christian. The most common strands are described below.

Roman Catholicism

Roman Catholicism is characterised by its doctrinal and organisational structure.

The Roman Catholic Church was first established by the Apostles, who followed Christ. Catholicism, which means universal, was described as 'Roman' by other Christian Churches. This was partly because of the Church's adoption of the organisational grid of the Roman Empire and partly because Saint Peter founded the Church in Rome, where subsequently he and Saint Paul were buried.

About half of the world's Christians are Roman Catholics. The Roman Catholic Church is led by the Pope. Roman Catholics believe that the Pope derives his authority in direct descent from St Peter, whom Jesus appointed as the leader of the Apostles.

Roman Catholics recognise the *New Testament* and the *Old Testament* (the Hebrew scriptures of Judaism). As well as the scriptures, the Catholic Church recognises other texts that are not recognised by Protestants. These are known by the Catholics as *Deuterocanonicals* and by Protestants as the *Apocrypha*. The emphasis of the faith is on prayer and the seven sacraments (baptism, penance, confirmation, the Eucharist, holy orders, matrimony, and the anointing of the sick). The Eucharist commemorates Christ's Last Supper by the consecration of bread and wine.

Protestantism

Protestantism grew out of a movement to reform the Catholic, or universal, church. It emphasised ways in which Christians should communicate with God, by reducing ritual and placing less importance on the role of the priest.

Although Protestantism started in Western Europe, it has spread to almost every nation. There are now several branches of the Protestant Church, including Lutherans, Baptists, Methodists, the Society of Friends and the Salvation Army.

Anglicanism

The Anglican Church is a worldwide group of independent churches that come under the Church of England. It was established in 1534 by King Henry VIII, who took control of the Church of England away from the Roman Catholic Pope. In 1549, Archbishop Thomas Cranmer recast many Roman Catholic texts into the Anglican *Book of Common Prayer*. Today, the Anglican Church embraces a diverse range of Christian faiths, from elements of Roman Catholicism to the newer Evangelical Churches. In this respect, the Anglican Church acts as a bridge between the Roman Catholic Church and the Protestant Churches. In recent times the Church of England has proved to be revisionist. For example, after much debate and internal conflict among its members, it has admitted women to the priesthood. In some cases this has led to entire congregations joining the Roman Catholic Church in protest.

The Orthodox Church

The Orthodox Church has no single leader analogous to the Pope, although it is led in each country by a senior archbishop called a Patriarch. The Orthodox Church exists in Greek and Russian forms and places great emphasis on tradition. All Orthodox services are rich in presentation and involve singing and bells, with incense, candles and glowing icons.

Worship

God is worshipped in three forms: the Father, the Son and the Holy Spirit (collectively, the Trinity). Although Christians have built churches since the end of the third century, they can worship anywhere. Services in churches and cathedrals are conducted by trained and ordained priests.

Diet

At one time Roman Catholics would not eat meat on a Friday. More recently this restriction has been lifted. However, restrictions regarding eating meat still apply to all Roman Catholics on Ash Wednesday and Good Friday.

Although restrictions on the diet of Roman Catholics on Friday have been relaxed, it is important to consider that older Roman Catholics may still wish to adhere strictly to these rules. It would be usual for them to eat fish on a Friday. Fish is also a suitable alternative to meat on Ash Wednesday and Good Friday.

Dress code

Christians generally wear the dress that is most commonly worn in the country in which they live.

QUESTIONS

?

Question 2

a. Where was Protestantism started?

_____

_____

b. What should Catholics not eat on a Friday?

_____

_____

Hinduism

Hinduism is the dominant religion of India, where approximately 80 per cent of the population are Hindu. It is about 3,500 years old.

In Britain, Hindus comprise 20 per cent of the South Asian population and are predominantly from the state of Gujarat in India, with a smaller number from the Punjab. It is estimated that there are about 360,000 Hindus in the UK.

Variations in Hindu practice depend on their country of origin. Some variations are also due to the interpretation of philosophies and scriptures by different Gurus (religious leaders). For example, the *skon* (*Hare Krishna*) movement has certain practices that are not followed by the majority of Hindus.

The basic premise of Hinduism is that it has no dogmatic creed and its worship has no fixed form. What makes or determines a Hindu rests on the fact that Hinduism is a way of life rather than a form of thought.

Hindus believe that *Parabrahma* is the supreme spirit of all creation. This spirit is perfect and unchanging and is neither male nor female. Although there are hundreds of Hindu Gods, the three most important, known as the trinity, are:

○ *Brahma* – the creator, who created the Hindu Gods

○ *Vishnu* – the protector

○ *Shiva* – the destroyer

All of the Gods and Goddesses are seen as manifestations of the same God.

Karma and rebirth

Hindus believe that the soul of human beings must be cleansed of earthly sins before it can return to Brahma. A person's *karma* is formed by their good or bad actions, and by religious merit gained in each life. This karma dictates what a person will be in their next life. Very bad karma may lead to a person being reborn as an animal or insect. When the person's soul is pure enough it returns to the Spirit of Creation.

Worship

Hindu worship may take place in either the home (domestic) or the *mandir* (temple). The heart of the temple is the central shrine, the home of the chief divinity. In the *mandir* women usually sit with the younger children, separate from the men. On festival days small images of the chief divinity are taken out and paraded.

Hindus are encouraged to pray at dawn and dusk, but the actual time is not critical. Worship at temples is between 6.30 am and 8.00 am and 7.00 pm and 8.30 pm. Hindus must wash thoroughly and change their clothes before praying.

Diet

Most Hindus are strict vegetarians. Some Hindus may be vegans (they do not eat any meat, fish, eggs or dairy produce) and many will not eat onions or garlic.

The cow is the most sacred animal to Hindus and to kill a cow is one of the greatest religious crimes. The pig is considered to be unclean and so pork products are not eaten. Hindus may not accept food that has come into contact with meat or meat products. They may insist on eating only food that has been prepared at home. Fasting is common among Hindus. This usually lasts for a day. Devout and orthodox Hindus do not smoke tobacco or drink alcohol (this particularly applies to women).

Dress code

A Hindu woman wears a glass wedding bangle on getting married and this is removed only if the husband dies. Breaking or removing a wedding bangle is considered an extremely bad omen.

Married women wear a *thali* (which looks like a nugget) on a chain at all times. This is removed only when the husband dies. Married Hindu women also wear a small circular spot, known as a *bindi*, on their forehead.

After *puja* (worship) some Hindus (both men and women), wear a red mark on their forehead as a blessing from the Gods.

Many Hindu women wear the *sari*, which is worn over a short blouse and an underskirt. The midriff is usually left bare. Many Hindu men and women wear European clothes, other than during worship or on festival days.

Many Hindus will wear a *khanthi* (beaded necklace) and a *janoi* (a sacred thread that passes diagonally across the body from the shoulder to about waist height). It is put on at important religious ceremonies and should never be removed. Some Hindus (men and women) wear a religious talisman on a chain, as a protection from evil.

Caste system

Although the caste (class) system no longer officially exists in India, there are people who still continue to preserve the system. Nowadays, there is a greater degree of movement between all castes, and the occupational rules are less rigidly adhered to.

Naming system

The pattern of Hindu names is: a personal (first) name that usually indicates sex, followed by a middle name (commonly either the father's or husband's name). The last name is the family name, which is shared by all the members of one division of a caste (class). It therefore gives information about the social status and traditional occupation of the owner. A typically constructed male name is *Anand Kumar Gupta*. An equivalent female name is *Bimla Ram Desai*. As a reaction against the caste system, some Hindus use their middle name as their surname, for example *Anand Kumar*.

Language

Hindus from Gujarat generally speak either *Gujarati* or *Hindi*. A few speak *Punjabi* or *Kutchi*.

QUESTIONS

?

Question 3

a. What do the following words mean:

○ **Brahma**

○ **Vishnu**

○ **Shiva**

b. What is a typically constructed male name?

Islam

Followers of Islam are called Muslims. Mohammed (born in 571AD), the 'Prophet and Messenger', was commanded by Allah (the one Muslim God) to convey his message. Prophet means 'good person' and Messenger means 'carries a message from God'.

Islam is seen as the youngest of the world's great religions. However, many, if not most, of the followers of Islam believe that:

○ Islam existed before Mohammed was born

○ The origins of Islam date back to the creation of the world

○ Mohammed was the last of a series of prophets and messengers of God.

Muslim is an Arabic word that refers to individuals who submit themselves to the 'Will of God'. Muslims believe in one God, Allah. Their Holy Book is the *Quran*. The religious duties of Muslims are described in the *Five Pillars of Islam*:

○ To recite at least once during their lifetime the *shahadah* (the creed, 'God is one and only one supreme creator, and Mohammed is the Messenger of God'). Most Muslims will repeat this once a day.

○ To perform the *salat* (prayer) five times a day. This is recited while facing towards Mecca (from the UK this is south east). Prayers are said at dawn, early afternoon, mid-afternoon, after sunset and just before sleep.

○ To donate annually to charity.

○ To fast during the month of *Ramadan*. The period when Ramadan occurs differs from year to year as Islam follows the lunar calendar.

○ If economically and physically possible/practical, to make at least one *hajj* (pilgrimage) to Mecca (the Muslim holy city).

There are two main groupings of Islam: the *Sunni* and the *Shi'ite* (pronounced shee-ite). Both adhere to the same body of beliefs, but differ in community organisation and in theological and legal practices. Central to these differences is the Shi'ite belief that only the descendants of the prophet Mohammed may adopt the title and role of *imam* (religious leader), while the Sunni (who comprise 90 per cent of Muslims) choose the *imam* by consensus.

In London, an *imam* is a local religious leader who has been appointed by the community. The *imam* is not always a community leader.

Worship

The religious centre for Muslims is the mosque. Inside a mosque men and women must have no physical contact.

Ritual cleansing (*wudu*) of the hands, arms up to the elbows, feet, face and top of the head takes place before prayer. Shoes are removed and the head is covered with a cap. Prayers are said on a small mat facing south east (in the UK) towards the *Ka'ba* in Mecca. Friday is the Muslim Holy day and congregational prayers are said at the mosques.

Muslims do not represent God in any shape or form, although Muslim families may have pictures of the Holy *Ka'ba* and the Mosque of the Prophet at Medina. They also have copies of the *Quran* holy scriptures in their homes.

Shoes must be removed before entering a mosque; this may be waived in life-threatening situations.

Diet

The diet of Muslims has spiritual importance and pork and pork products are forbidden. Meat from other animals must have been ritually slaughtered in the correct manner to remove blood, which Muslims do not consume. This meat is known as *halal*.

In extreme circumstances Muslims may eat *kosher* food instead of halal. Kosher meat is prepared for Jewish people in a similar way to halal meat. However, this will probably be unacceptable to some Muslims from the Middle East. Alcohol is forbidden. Muslims do not eat shellfish.

Dress code

The high moral values of Islam require men and women to keep their bodies covered at all times from their faces down. This applies particularly when in public places. Many women will wear head scarves (*hijab*), especially inside the mosque.

Naming system

The Muslim naming format may vary according to the area from which an individual originates. All Muslims will be given a personal name and usually have two or more names.

Men

○ Men will first have a religious name such as *Mohammed*, *Allah* or *Amin*.

○ They will then have a personal name such as *Ahmed*, *Anwar*, *Arif*, *Hanif*, *Iqbal*, *Ishmael*, *Jabar*, *Malik*, *Nasim*, *Rashid* or *Yusuf*.

○ Examples of a male name would be *Mohammed Anwar* or *Akbar Malik*.

○ The personal name can be used alone, although it is more polite to use the religious and personal names together.

○ Some men will not have a religious name and will use two personal names instead. If this is the case, the second personal name may sometimes be used in the UK as a surname.

○ Muslim men originating from some areas of the world may have a family name. In Pakistan common family names are *Chaudrey* and *Khan*. In this case a man's name may consist of a religious name, a personal name and a family name, such as *Akbar Jamal Khan*.

○ When asking a Muslim for their first name it is inappropriate to ask them for their Christian name.

Women

Women will have a personal name such as *Amina*, *Fatima*, *Jameela*, *Nasreen*, *Razia* or *Yasmin*. They will also have a female title name such as *Begum*, *Bibi*, *Kanum* or *Khatoon*. Examples of a female name would be *Fatima Khatoon* or *Ayesha Bibi*.

It is important that a Muslim female is addressed either by her personal name only or formally by her personal and title name together. Never address her by her title name only. Some women may also have a family name.

QUESTIONS

?

Question 4

a. What is the name given to the head scarves that Muslim women wear?

_____

_____

b. What meat can a Muslim never eat?

_____

_____

Judaism

Judaism originated in the Middle East and dates back more than 4,000 years. Jewish people believe that a single transcendent God created the universe and continues providentially to govern it. This same God revealed himself to the Israelites at Mount Sinai. The content of that revelation is the *Torah* (revealed instruction). God's will for humankind is expressed in the Ten Commandments.

A second major concept of Judaism is the covenant, or contractual agreement, between God and the Jewish people. They would acknowledge God, agreeing to obey his law; God, in turn, would acknowledge Israelites as his chosen people.

Orthodox (strict) Jews believe that the Jewish laws and teachings of the *Torah* must be followed exactly as they were laid down in the time of Moses.

Non-orthodox or progressive Jews believe that some of the *Torah's* teachings may be adapted to make them more relevant to modern life. Progressive Jews are known by different names (for example Reform, Conservative and Liberal Jews), depending on which movement they follow.

Worship

The *synagogue* is a house of prayer and study as well as a community centre. Three prayer sessions are taken daily, although prayers can be said anywhere. Normally men, and sometimes women, come together for prayers. For communal prayer to take place it is necessary for a *minyan* to be present: a group of 10 adult male (progressives include female) Jews.

Most synagogues will have a Rabbi who can advise the community about the interpretation of religious laws. The Rabbi may lead the service and read a different part of the *Torah* each week. Although the Rabbi is usually the person leading the service, anybody who is able to may lead the service. All men must cover their heads when entering a synagogue.

Diet

Some Jews are very strict about following dietary laws (*kashrut*). Animals, birds and fish are either *kosher* (permitted) or *treif* (forbidden). Animals that chew the cud and have cloven hooves (such as cows, sheep and goats), all fowl (apart from birds of prey) and fish with fins and scales are kosher as long as they are prepared according to Jewish laws. Pork and shellfish are forbidden. Foods that contain or have been cooked in forbidden products are also unacceptable.

Orthodox Jews will not eat milk and meat products together on the same plate or at the same time. Separate sets of utensils are kept for cooking meat and dairy dishes. Utensils used for dairy products are washed in a separate sink from those used for meat dishes. Some orthodox Jews may wait for several hours after eating a meat dish before eating a milk product. Fruit and vegetables are eaten.

Dress code

Some orthodox Jewish men keep their heads covered at all times, usually with a *kippah* (skull cap). Some observant married women cover their heads with hats, scarves or wigs when in public. No observant woman will wear sleeveless dresses, miniskirts or trousers. For morning prayer and on the evening of the Day of Atonement, Jewish men wear prayer shawls. They also wear *phylacteries* (small leather boxes containing Biblical texts) on their forehead and left upper arm. Male *Hasidim* and members of some other ultra orthodox sects wear dark clothes, long coats and wide-brimmed hats.

Naming system

Jewish families usually take the naming system of the country in which they live. Most married women take their husband's name. Jewish people may also have a Hebrew name, which may appear on their Hebrew marriage certificate (*katuba*) and on their tombstone above their British name.

QUESTIONS

?

Question 5

What do the following words mean?

○ Kashrut

○ Kosher

○ Treif

○ Kippah

Sikhism

The Sikh religion, a modern, democratic, versatile and young religion, was founded by Guru Nanak (1469–1538), who was born in the village Talwandi, now called Nanakana Sahib, near Lahore (Pakistan). Guru Nanak and the Nine Gurus who succeeded him set an example of living spiritually while taking an active part in the secular world. The teachings and the divine message of the Ten Gurus, enshrined in the *Guru Granth Sahib* (one of the highly respected Holy books), was written and compiled by the Gurus themselves and recorded in the *Granth Sahib*.

The definition of a Sikh

The word sikh means disciple or student. Any human being who faithfully believes in the following and does not owe allegiance to any other religion is a Sikh:

❍ One immortal being

❍ Ten Gurus, from Guru Nanak Sahib to Guru Gobind Singh Sahib

❍ The *Guru Granth Sahib*

❍ The utterances and teachings of the Ten Gurus

❍ Khande di Pahual (the baptism ceremony) bequeathed by the tenth Guru.

The tenth Guru, Guru Gobind Singh (1666–1708), initiated the Sikh baptism ceremony (*Amrit*) on 30 March 1699. Baptised Sikhs are called *Khalsa* (God's own). The initiation day of the Sikhs' baptism is called *Vaisakhi Day*, meaning the birth of Khalsa; hence, this day has a significant religious importance for Sikhs all over the world. The Sikhs acquired their religious uniform, consisting of the Five Ks, on this day.

Sikhism emphasises the truth and creativity of a personal God and urges union with him through meditation and surrender to his will. Sikhs do not believe in the worship of idols, or rituals. Gods and Goddesses are considered non-entities. The religion embraces practical living, rendering service to humanity and engendering tolerance and love to all. It is estimated that there are more than 300,000 Sikhs in the UK, which would make this the largest Sikh community in any country outside India.

Sikhs conform to a code of conduct called the *Sikh Rahit Marayada*. This code of conduct forbids them from:

○ Cutting or trimming their hair

○ Cohabiting with a person other than one's spouse

○ Consuming intoxicants such as drugs, tobacco and alcohol

○ Eating *halal* or *kosher* meat

○ Worshipping idols or icons.

Worship

Sikhs worship in a gurdwara (*gur-dwa-ra*, from the word *gurudwara* meaning place of worship). Sikhs would be offended if the gurdwara was searched without first consulting community leaders and gurdwara officials. A triangular orange flag indicates that an otherwise ordinary building is a gurdwara.

Sikhs worship every day – mornings and evenings. Working families may attend the gurdwara only on Sundays, the only convenient or common day for them.

A large room in the gurdwara containing the *Sri Guru Granth Sahib* (Holy Book) is used for prayer and worship. Worshippers and visitors alike must remove their shoes and cover their heads prior to entering this room.

Gurdwaras are not all identical but certain features are always present; in particular, they all have the dais (*takht*), from which the Holy Book is read, with a whisk (*chaur*) and a canopy above it (wherever the Holy Book is displayed, even in houses, it will have a canopy above it). Women play an active and equal role in all gurdwara worship. They may conduct services, read from the Holy Book in public and vote on all matters related to the running and function of the gurdwara.

Sikhs are renowned for their hospitality. Apart from being a place of worship and a house for the *Sri Guru Granth Sahib*, the gurdwara is also a guesthouse where passing travellers may find free food (*Langar*) and shelter during their stay.

Diet

Sikhs must not eat meat that has been killed in a ritualistic manner. This prohibits the eating of *halal* and *kosher* meat. All baptised Sikhs are vegetarians, although there is no restriction for the consumption of meat. Sikhs who do eat meat must only eat *chatka* meat, from animals that have been killed quickly, humanely and without religious or ritual ceremonies.

Dress code

Women dress modestly. Traditionally they wear loose trousers (*shalwar*), a long tunic (*kameez*) and a long scarf (*chuni*) to cover the head as a mark of respect, to elders and especially when in the gurdwara.

Most men will wear western clothes when in public. At home they may wear loose-fitting cotton trousers with a long overshirt. Sikh men will wear a turban as soon as they are old enough (usually at the age of 13 or 14). Generally, the colour of the turban has no particular significance and is a matter of personal choice.

The Five Ks are: *kangah* (a small wooden comb); *kacha* (similar to shorts); *kara* (a steel bracelet); *kirpan* (a small ceremonial sword in a shoulder belt); *kesh* (long uncut and untrimmed hair and beard).

The five Ks explained

Kangah (miniature comb) A small comb, either of wood or plastic, to help keep the hair clean. It is usually kept tucked into the hair bun of men and tucked into the back of the head (either over or under the plait) of women. Some combs may have a little knife embedded in them.

Kacha (shorts) A pair of shorts (similar to boxer shorts) reminds Sikhs that it is prohibited to cohabit with a person other than one's spouse. They're worn at all times and can be worn under trousers or on their own.

Kara (steel bangle) A steel bangle to remind a Sikh to abstain from the act of theft. Very thick karas are often seen worn by some Sikhs, although these are not clearly defined. A kara is usually the first visible sign of a Sikh.

Kirpan (knife) A steel knife (mini sword) for self-defence (only to be used as a last resort) to instill the spirit of self-respect and sense of freedom from oppression. Baptised Sikh men and women wear it at all times either under or outside their clothing. The full-size sword is usually reserved for ceremonial and religious purposes.

Kesh (hair) Natural hair growth; uncut and untrimmed hair (part of the Sikh uniform) is a mark of saintly appearance and complete submission to the Will of God who gave this physical form to the human race. It can be of any length, but must be sheathed.

Naming system

The Sikh name is usually in three parts, but for religious reasons most Sikhs in India no longer use the third part, i.e. the family surname (instead they use their father's name, i.e. son of…). In the UK, however, more and more Sikhs are beginning to use the last name.

First names can be common to both sexes. The second name will either be Singh (meaning *lion*) for a man or Kaur (meaning *princess*) for a woman. A family name follows the first and second names. Those who do not use a family name may adopt Singh or Kaur (instead of their father's name) as their surname, and will then be correctly addressed as Mr and Mrs Singh or Mrs, Ms, Miss Kaur.

Language

The mother tongue of Sikhs is Punjabi (derived from the words *punj ab*, meaning five rivers). Punjab is located in the North West of the subcontinent amongst the famous five rivers, hence land of five rivers

Question 6

a. What does the word Sikh mean?

_____

_____

b. Where do Sikhs worship?

_____

_____

SECTION 2: Culture and communities

African-Caribbeans

The term African-Caribbean reflects the fact that most people from the Caribbean are descendants of people transported from their homes in West Africa to work as slaves in the West Indies on the cotton, sugar and tobacco plantations.

Not all people from the Caribbean islands are of African descent. After the slave trade was abolished by parliament in 1807, and slavery in the British Caribbean ended in 1834, people from India and China were recruited as indentured labour to work on the plantations.

Many African-Caribbean men arrived in the UK during the Second World War to work in the munitions factories, the Merchant Navy or the Armed Services. With the reconstruction of the UK after the Second World War, there were huge labour shortages in the transport industry and the National Health Service (NHS). Many African-Caribbean workers were recruited from the Caribbean islands with promises of a higher standard of living in the UK, to fill the labour-scarce sectors of industry.

About 60 per cent of African-Caribbeans who migrated to the UK originated in Jamaica. Other African-Caribbeans have origins in islands such as Barbados, Dominica, Trinidad, St Lucia and St Vincent.

Religion

Although most major religions of the world are to be found in the Caribbean islands, Christianity is the predominant religion among the British African-Caribbean community. Many are more active in non-traditionalist churches and Christian revivalist movements, such as the Pentecostal Church.

Language

By the mid-1700s every Caribbean island was controlled by a European country. Consequently, the most commonly spoken languages throughout the Caribbean islands are English, French and Spanish.

The names given to individuals are diverse and depend upon the island from which an individual's family originates. English names were generally given on many of the British controlled islands. These names sometimes reflect those of famous English citizens, but are more usually similar to those of the white British population. Other names have Asian, Dutch and French origins such as:

○ Asian: Kanhai, Patel, Singh

○ Dutch: Eickhof, Maartens

○ French: François, Pierre

Question 7

a. What is the predominant religion amongst the British African–Caribbean community?

_____

_____

b. What is the most common language spoken throughout the Caribbean islands?

_____

Arabs

Arabs may be described as those people who originate from North Africa and the Middle East (from Western Morocco to Oman in the East and from Turkey in the North to Yemen and Sudan in the South). The Arab heartland is _Hijaz_ (now Western Saudi Arabia).

A popular misconception is that Arab identity is determined by religion and that if you are Muslim you are an Arab. This is not so. For example, the nation of Iran is composed of Muslims who are Persians, not Arabs. Likewise Indonesia, the world's most populous Muslim nation, is inhabited by Malays, not Arabs. Many British Muslims originate from non-Arabic countries, such as Pakistan and Somalia. There are also Christian Arabs throughout the Middle East.

Religion

More than 85 per cent of all Arabs are Sunni Muslims, and ten per cent are Shi'ite Muslims (located around Yemen, Iraq and the Gulf Coast). Fewer than five per cent are Christians, who generally live in Egypt, Lebanon, Syria, Palestine, Jordan and Israel.

Dress code

Traditional Arab male dress is a long-sleeved dress that covers the whole body and is called a _dishdashah_ or _thoub_. This garment is intended to keep the body cool by allowing air to circulate.

Men also wear a three-piece head cover. The bottom piece is a white cap (_thagiyah_), which is used to keep the hair in place. On top of the _thagiyah_ is a scarf-like head cover: a light version for summer (_gutrah_) and a heavier red-and-white checked version worn in winter (_shumag_). The head covers are held in place by a black band called an _ogal_. Boys begin to wear the head cover upon reaching puberty as a sign of entering manhood. The head covering is not worn inside the home unless guests are present. In the UK many Arab men now wear western clothes.

Most Arab women dress conservatively, covering their faces and hair. Often they wear a long black garment called an _abayah_, which covers the body from the shoulders to the feet. This can be worn over either a traditional Arabian dress or the latest international fashion. More conservative women and girls may wear a face and head cover; others may wear a scarf-like cover called a _hijab_ that covers the hair, but not the face

Language

The spoken and written language of the Arab people is Arabic.

QUESTIONS

?

Question 8

a. What is the name given to traditional Arab male dress?

_____

_____

b. What is the spoken and written language of the Arab people?

_____

_____

Bangladeshis

Bangladeshis originate from Bangladesh, known as East Pakistan before gaining independence from Pakistan in 1971. East Pakistan had originally been carved out of the Indian State of Bengal when British India was partitioned into the two states of India and Pakistani in 1947. Today, Bangladesh shares a border with the Indian State of West Bengal, whose inhabitants are also Bengali.

The first Bangladeshis arrived in the UK in the early 1950s. Many came from Sylhet, a rural district in the north east that has strong links with the UK and its colonial past. Historically, many of the men worked as merchant seamen

Religion

Bangladeshis are predominantly Muslims.

Diet

The staple diet of Bangladeshis is rice, fish and curry. Many Bangladeshis also eat meat. Bangladeshis are Muslims and are not permitted to eat pork. All other meat is acceptable, provided it is _halal_.

Dress code

Bangladeshi women may wear Muslim dress or a _sari_, which is worn over a short blouse and an underskirt. It would be unusual for the midriff to be left bare. Some women may wear a _shalwarkameez_ (loose-fitting trousers and long shirt).

Language

The official language of Bangladesh and the language most commonly spoken by Bangladeshis is Bengali. British Bangladeshis speak the Sylhet dialect of Bengali (known as Bangla or Sylheti). Among older Bangladeshis, Bengali is still the principal language of communication. Younger Bangladeshis are more likely to speak English. Today, at least 40 per cent of the Bangladeshi community in the UK is aged under 20 years.

QUESTIONS

Question 9

a. Where do Bangladeshis originate?

_____

_____

b. What religion are Bangladeshis?

_____

_____

Chinese

The latter half of the 19th century and the beginning of the 20th century saw large numbers of Chinese emigrate to many parts of the world in search of work, a number of them as indentured labourers. Migration to the UK began in the early 19th century with the arrival of Chinese sailors, who settled in the major port areas of Bristol, Cardiff, Liverpool and London.

In the late 1950s and throughout the 1960s and 1970s large numbers of Chinese migrated to the UK from the New Territories of Hong Kong. Today, more than a third of the UK's Chinese community originates from Hong Kong.

Other East Asians originate from Vietnam (having arrived as political refugees at the end of the Vietnam War and as 'boat people' in the late 1970s as a result of China's war with Vietnam), Malaysia, the Philippines and Singapore. Political unrest in recent decades in China, such as the Cultural Revolution in the 1970s and the Democracy Movement in the 1980s, has also led to Chinese nationals seeking political asylum in the UK and other Western countries.

Chinese settlement in the UK tends to have been more scattered than that of other ethnic minorities, due primarily to their involvement in the catering trade (although many second and third generation Chinese are now employed in a wide range of professions).

Religion

The principal religions practised in China are Buddhism, Confucianism and Taoism (pronounced Daoism).

Some Chinese are Roman Catholics or Protestants, and significant minorities in China also practise Islam and Hinduism.

Although Confucianism is a social philosophy, some Chinese practise it as a form of worship. However, the second and third generations are less likely to observe the doctrine than the first generation.

Naming system

The family name can be regarded as the surname for British purposes. For example:

Female

❍ _Yeung_ (family name)

❍ _Lan-Ying_ (personal name)

Male

○ *Xu* (family name)

○ *Nai-Gang* (personal name)

Examples of the more common Chinese names found in the UK are *Chang*, *Cheung*, *Lam*, *Lee*, *Leung*, *Man* and *Wong*. It is usual for a wife and children to take the husband's family name. For example: *Lee May-Lin* would become *Yeung Lee May-Lin*. Many Chinese follow the British naming system, giving their family name last. For example: *Nai-Gang Xu*.

The Chinese may use a European name as well, which they will give with their family name, e.g. *Wendy Chang*.

It is polite to check which naming system a Chinese person uses. Children usually use the father's family name. The wife may retain her maiden name, in which case she will refer to herself as Ms. If she uses her husband's family name she will refer to herself as Mrs. It is not unusual for married Chinese women to use both maiden and married names interchangeably.

The use of nicknames in the Chinese community is widespread – so much so that long-term acquaintances may know each other only by their nicknames.

Language

The official language of China is Mandarin, although a variety of other dialects is also spoken. In the Southern Chinese province of Kwangtung, Cantonese is the principal language, and this is also spoken in Hong Kong and Macau. Cantonese is therefore the language predominantly used by the majority of the UK's Chinese population. Those who have emigrated from Singapore and Malaysia are more likely to speak Mandarin.

QUESTIONS

Question 10

a. What are the principal languages spoken in China?

....

....

b. What is the official language of China?

....

....

Gypsies and travellers

The traditional gypsy and traveller populations in the UK originate from two separate ethnic groups. These consist of indigenous nomadic groups, identified in records dating back to the 12th century (of whom Irish travellers currently form the largest) and the Roma Gypsies, whose ancestors originated in North West India and moved gradually across Persia and the Middle East into Europe, first arriving in the UK in the 15th century, and more recently coming as refugees from Eastern Europe, in particular the former Yugoslavia.

Gypsies and Irish Travellers are recognised under the Race Relations Amendment Act 2000, together with other indigenous nomadic groups such as Scottish and Welsh Travellers.

Non-traditional or New Travellers are not recognised as an ethnic group but, for the purposes of site provision, trespass and education, the law treats them the same and they experience many of the same problems.

Discrimination

Gypsies and travellers have suffered discrimination and persecution over many centuries. Examples include the death penalty for being a gypsy in the reign of Elizabeth I, enslavement until the 19th century in many parts of Europe and persecution by the Nazis during the Second World War.

It is not uncommon to hear gypsies and travellers publicly referred to in racist terms in a way that would be totally unacceptable for any other ethnic group. The need to survive and to protect their self-esteem has led gypsies and travellers to keep themselves separate from mainstream society and its institutions and to view outsiders with suspicion.

Nomadism

The nomadic way of life was based on economic necessity, so gypsies and travellers provided what was not readily available in small, dispersed communities – music, metal work, a variety of hardware and small luxuries, and skilled casual labour in agricultural areas. Gypsies and travellers have moved into cities for the same economic reasons as the settled population. Strong and distinctive cultures have grown up, very much based on self-reliance and family connections. Although gypsies and indigenous travellers are distinct ethnic groups there are many parallels in their cultures deriving from their nomadic life-style and how they have been marginalised by society. In the UK the majority of gypsies and travellers are no longer nomadic, often because of the shortage of caravan site provision. Those who are on the road are those who have failed to get on an official site, and cannot cope with going into housing. Gypsies and travellers who no longer travel still perceive themselves as belonging to their cultural group.

Gypsies

Sometimes called Romanies or Romani, UK gypsies are part of a worldwide ethnic minority originating from India. Gypsies are the largest ethnic minority in continental Europe, but form a small, dispersed population in the UK. The UK gypsy community originally spoke a dialect of Romani, but now speaks a variety of English using Romani words.

Other information

Taboos and rituals connected with water and cleanliness are part of the gypsy heritage and are still adhered to by more traditional gypsies. Water remains important for many gypsies and travellers on the road as it is sometimes difficult to access.

Irish traveller

Irish travellers are often dismissed as not being 'real' gypsies and therefore suffer a double discrimination. This could mean they are not allowed to put their name down for a pitch on an official site.

Irish travellers have become more assertive in claiming their cultural heritage, which has been difficult as lack of literacy leaves them with no written records of their own and they are a far smaller group than gypsies. Suffice to say that there are records going back at least 700 years of a distinct, separate, nomadic group using their own language, moving backwards and forwards to Ireland and working as metal workers, hence the name 'Tinkers'.

Irish travellers are all members of the Roman Catholic Church and hold very strong traditional beliefs on such issues as marriage and divorce. Early marriage is very common and young women are not allowed to go out alone until they are married.

Issues arising from poor levels of literacy and the use of dogs are shared with the gypsy community.

Roma refugees

The Roma population of Eastern Europe has been systematically repressed under the Communist regimes (with the exception of Tito's Yugoslavia). Their Roma language was forbidden, they couldn't travel and many were forced to live in ghettos. The demise of the Iron Curtain does not appear to have relieved the situation, and many have fled to Western Europe to escape physical attacks, victimisation and harassment.

When they arrive in the UK many Roma experience prejudice and disadvantage on the basis both of being asylum seekers and of being gypsies. Few speak English. There are few Roma interpreters and the home countries' interpreters (Czech, Serb and Romanian) are often deeply prejudiced against them.

They have in common with all gypsies and travellers the fact that they have been marginalised, which means that they generally lack formal education.

New travellers

These are a very diverse group ranging from well organised groups who are ideologically committed to a sustainable way of life, and often hold down professional jobs, to groups of young people and young families who are there because of limited choices in their lives. A local survey undertaken by The Children's Society has shown that a significant number of 'New Travellers' are young people who have left care or are escaping poor housing or difficult home situations.

Some 'New Travellers' are now second and third generation on the road and travel in family groups in much the same style as traditional travellers.

Indian

India was, with Pakistan and Bangladesh, part of British India until it was granted independence on 14 August, 1947. India is made up of 22 states and nine union territories, which are each separate administrative entities with their own defined powers and responsibilities. Each of these states demonstrates diversity in language, religion and culture. South Asians may differ in religion, culture and nationality through their national origins in Bangladesh, Pakistan or India, and Indians are equally diverse. Many British Indians originate from Gujarat and are mainly Hindus. The UK first established links with Gujarat when the British East India Company set up its first trading post on the Gujarat coast in the 17th century. The 19th century saw the first Gujaratis arrive in the UK as students. The most famous of these, a law student, Mohandas Gandhi, later led India to independence and became known as 'Mahatma' (noble hearted). Following the labour shortages after the Second World War, the British government encouraged immigrants from Gujarat to come to the UK, bringing with them their experience of the steel and textile industries. Another group came from Uganda as refugees in 1971, expelled by the dictator Idi Amin. The majority of Punjabis now living in the UK are Sikhs. One reason for Sikhs coming to the UK is their historical connection with the British Armed Forces, with many of them having served during the Second World War.

Religion

About 85 per cent of the population of India is Hindu, about 10 per cent is Muslim and the rest of the population is made up of Christians, Sikhs, Buddhists and Jews.

Dress code

South Asian women of all the religions of India traditionally wear the *sari*, which is worn over a short blouse and an underskirt. The midriff is usually left bare. The *shalwar kameez*, though traditionally Sikh dress, is now being worn very widely by other groups.

Married Hindu women also wear a small circular spot, known as a *bindi*, on their forehead. The *bindi* is usually red, but these days may be different colours and not only restricted to Hindus.

Language

There are more than 15 major languages used throughout India and more than 500 different dialects. The most common languages are Hindi, Urdu, Punjabi and Gujarati.

QUESTIONS

?

Question 12

a. When was India granted independence?

_____

_____

b. What are the most common Indian languages?

_____

_____

Irish

The 1991 census showed that 592,550 Irish born in the Irish Republic and 244,914 Irish born in Northern Ireland were resident in the UK. London accounts for 36 per cent of those from the Irish Republic and 17 per cent of those from Northern Ireland. Irish people make up the largest and longest established resident minority ethnic community in the UK. Irish immigrants and their descendants represent 10 per cent of the London population.

The first settlers from Ireland began to arrive in London towards the end of the 12th century, following the Anglo-Norman invasion of Ireland. However, the number of Irish people in Britain remained fairly low until the economic turmoil of the early 19th century led many rural labourers and farmers to emigrate to Britain. Emigration to Britain from Ireland culminated in mass migration between 1847 and 1848 during the Great Potato Famine when more than 800,000 people are believed to have died. It is estimated that by 1851 more than 100,000 Irish were living in London, where they accounted for about one in 20 of the population. In fact, the relationship between Britain and Ireland is the longest that either country has shared with another.

Immigration into the UK from Ireland slowed during the 1960s as a result of an economic boom in Ireland. However, by the 1980s rising unemployment in Ireland led to many young Irish once more heading for London. Today, more people migrate from the UK to Ireland than vice versa.

Religion

Most members of the Irish community who originate from Ireland are Catholic. Nonetheless, care must be taken not to make assumptions about which religion an Irish person practises, as religion is a very sensitive issue. Irish people from Northern Ireland may be Catholic, Protestant or Presbyterian. People from Northern Ireland who are Anglican, Catholic or Presbyterian may not identify themselves as Irish.

Language

Both Gaelic and English are spoken in Ireland. Most members of the Irish community will speak English.

QUESTIONS

Question 13

a. Why did the Irish people emigrate to Britain between 1847–1848?

_____

_____

b. What two languages are spoken in Ireland?

_____

_____

Japanese

The British Japanese community is fairly new compared to other communities. In London, as British–Japanese business ties have grown, more Japanese business men and women have taken up residence. At the same time, this growth in business relations has led to many young Japanese coming to the UK to study.

Religion

The Japanese may follow either or both the Shinto and Buddhist religions. When Buddhism was first introduced to Japan in the 6th century, the Shinto and Buddhist beliefs began to interact. When events are associated with community festivals or some religious activity, they are usually celebrated at a local Shinto shrine. This is because the rites that accompany a person throughout their life are usually associated with Shinto. Buddhism, being concerned with the continuing life cycle, tends to be associated with death and the memorial of family members.

Shinto is associated with the mythology of Japan's creation and the supernatural ancestors of Japan's imperial line. It is the foundation of Japan's identity as a nation. Shinto is concerned with notions of pollution and purity; washing on entry to a shrine purifies a person from the pollution of the outside world and marks the sacred inside of the shrine compound.

Two other religions that have had a significant impact on Japanese society and culture are Confucianism and Taoism.

Language

The official language of Japan is Japanese.

QUESTIONS

?

Question 13

a. What two religions might the Japanese follow?

_____

_____

b. What is the official language of Japan?

_____

_____

Kosovans

Kosovo was once part of the Turkish Empire, but anti-Turkish resistance succeeded in expelling the Turks and Kosovo became part of the newly founded state of Albania in 1912. However, in the following year the great European powers, including Britain, forced Albania to relinquish Kosovo to Serbia, which itself was incorporated into the new Kingdom of Yugoslavia in 1918.

After the Second World War, Kosovo was granted autonomy within Serbia and this autonomy grew as a result of pressure and riots from the ethnic Albanian population. Riots in 1981 incited a Serbian backlash and increased Serbian resentment of Albanians. This led to the rise of power of the Serbian nationalist Slobodan Milosevic. The Albanian media were suppressed, all Albanian language education was halted and the autonomous Kosovan parliament was abolished in 1990.

In 1998/9 Serb militias, extremist groups from Belgrade and paramilitary units drove Muslims from their homes in carefully planned operations, which were known as 'ethnic cleansing'. The situation became so serious that in early 1999 NATO forces launched an air campaign to force the withdrawal of all Serbian military personnel from the province. Hundreds of thousands of Kosovo Albanians fled to neighbouring countries.

Following Serbian withdrawal from the province in 1999, Kosovo is once again an autonomous region of Serbia under the present governance of an international peacekeeping force, KFOR (Kosovo Force). Although many of the Kosovar Albanian refugees have now returned home, Kosovo remains a dangerous place, with ethnic conflict still an everyday occurrence. Many Kosovar Albanian refugees remain in the UK, too frightened to return home.

Religion

The majority of Kosovar Albanians are Muslim, although they are not strict. The older generations tend to be more orthodox, although they are still less likely to be as orthodox as other Muslims.

Many younger Kosovar Albanians are not strict about their diet and will eat meat that is not *halal*. This may differ among Kosovar Albanians who have originated from more rural areas. To the older, more orthodox generations of Kosovar Albanians the issue of whether or not meat is *halal* may be more important.

Language

Most Kosovans speak Albanian.

QUESTIONS

Question 14

a. Kosovo was once part of which empire?

b. What is the main religion of Kosovo?

The lesbian, gay and bisexual community

The following information highlights issues in relation to the lesbian, gay and bisexual (LGB) community. It is recognised, however, that many of the experiences of discrimination, victimisation and harassment affecting lesbians, gay men and bisexuals also apply to transgender people. Because of these links, a number of organisations have emerged in recent years that represent lesbian, gay, bisexual *and* transgender communities (including the LGBTAG).

London is home to a large and diverse population of lesbian, gay men, and bisexuals, many having moved here from rural communities, small towns and other countries hoping to find a more welcoming environment. A survey conducted by *Gay Times* in 1997 estimated that there were over 600 LGB commercial venues such as bars and restaurants and more than 1100 community groups in the UK.

It is estimated that LGBs make up around 10 per cent of the UK population (although it is difficult to provide more accurate statistics because at present information on the number of lesbians, gay men and bisexuals resident in the UK is not recorded in the national census).

Coming out

Coming out describes the process whereby a lesbian, gay or bisexual person tells someone, publicly or privately, that they are LGB. Many LGB people are not out, often because of a fear of violence, ridicule or harassment from family, friends or work colleagues.

Young people are often attacked or evicted from their family homes when they tell family members that they are lesbian, gay or bisexual. Many face violence and homophobic bullying at school and on the street. LGB adults may already have endured years of keeping an important part of their lives and identities secret. Coming out may result in losing contact with parents, children, friends, community and work associates.

Even when a member of the lesbian, gay or bisexual community is out, it does not mean they are out to everyone. They may have told family members or friends and not told work colleagues or associates. Conversely, they may have told work colleagues but not family and friends.

The most significant people in their lives (parents, for example) are often the last to be told. This may be linked to an individual's negative frame of reference about being lesbian, gay or bisexual, formed by social and domestic pressures to conform to the majority 'heterosexual' group.

There are many myths and stereotypes associated with the LGB community, and we should seek to question and challenge them wherever possible. The following are typical examples: *Lesbians are masculine and gay men are effeminate*: the reality is that LGB people express their femininity or masculinity no differently from heterosexual men and women. *Gay men are likely to be HIV positive*: the reality is that infection rates of HIV are higher among the heterosexual community than among the gay community and that, proportionately, gay men are no more likely to be HIV positive than heterosexual men and women.

Family life

Many lesbians, gay men and bisexuals are in committed long-term relationships. It is important to be aware of different family structures and recognise that not all families are representative of the traditional family structure. For example, some children may have same-sex parents. Children raised within LGB families often have extended family members who are also part of the lesbian, gay or bisexual community. A common myth is that a child from an LGB family is likely to grow up to be lesbian, gay or bisexual or may be disadvantaged by not being brought up by parents from both sexes. This is unfounded and recent research indicates that children who grow up in LGB families are just as healthy, balanced and well cared for as those brought up within a more traditional family structure.

Some communities, cultures and religions in the UK hold strong beliefs about 'traditional family life' and LGB issues. Faced with these circumstances, some LGB people who remain in traditional family structures may never reveal or acknowledge that they are lesbian, gay or bisexual. They have little choice but to conform to the perceived traditional values expected by their families, friends, work colleagues and other associates.

Terminology

○ *Bisexual*, someone who is attracted to both sexes emotionally and/or physically.

○ *Closet* (as in 'in the closet'), an individual's choice not to tell others that they are gay, lesbian or bisexual.

○ *Out* (as in coming out), to tell other people, publicly or privately that one is lesbian, gay or bisexual.

○ *Heterosexual* or 'straight', someone who is attracted, emotionally and/or physically to the opposite sex.

○ *Homosexual*, medical term used to criminalise lesbians, gay men and bisexuals in the 19th century. The term should generally be avoided, although some older LGB people may describe themselves in this way.

- *Lesbian*, a woman who is attracted emotionally and/or physically to other women.

- *Polaris*, secret language developed in the 1950s and 1960s to allow lesbians, gay men and bisexuals to communicate discreetly in public. Aspects of the language are still in use today.

- *Queer bashing*, violent stranger attacks on lesbians, gay men and bisexuals, or those who are perceived to be.

- *Rent boy*, a young male who sells sex to other men. Not always gay.

- *Scene* (as in 'gay scene'), commercial venues where LGB people socialise. Mainly pubs and clubs.

- *Sexuality/sexual orientation*, terms often used in relation to LGB issues.

QUESTIONS

?

Quetion 15

What do the following words mean?

- Bisexual

- Heterosexual

Pakistan

The modern state of Pakistan (formerly West Pakistan) was created in 1947 as a result of the partition of British India along religious lines. West Pakistan was defined by drawing a dividing line through Kashmir, thereby separating it from India and recognising that the majority of West Pakistan's population was Muslim and that of India was predominantly Hindu. A civil war in 1971 led to East Pakistan seceding from Pakistan to become Bangladesh. West Pakistan became known as Pakistan.

The division of Kashmir was bitterly opposed by both India and Pakistan at the time and has remained a source of tension and conflict. Many early Pakistani settlers arrived in Britain from the Mirpur region of the Punjab in the early 1890s. Others settled after the Second World War, having served in the British Armed Forces. Encouraged by the British government, further immigrants from Pakistan arrived in the 1950s and 1960s, to assist with Britain's post-war reconstruction.

Religion

Pakistan was created for the majority followers of Islam (Muslims) who inhabited the area. To that extent, Islam dictates the life and culture of the Pakistani people.

Dress code

Pakistani women traditionally wear the *salwar kameez* (loose trousers and a long tunic). It is unusual for the midriff to be left bare. Many also wear a *sari* over a short blouse and an underskirt. Some women wear traditional long dresses and cover their heads with a scarf (*hijab*).

Language

The official language of Pakistan is Urdu, although Sindhi, Pashto and Punjabi are also spoken. The majority of people from Pakistan will, however, speak Urdu or Punjabi.

QUESTIONS

Question 16

a. When was the state of Pakistan created?

_____

_____

b. What is the official language of Pakistan?

_____

_____

Somalis

Somalis originate from Somalia, located on the Horn of Africa. The Somalis or Samaal consist of six major clan-families. Four of the families represent about 70 per cent of Somalia's population. These are the _Dir_, _Daarood_, _Isaaq_ and _Hawiye_ families who originally led a predominantly pastoral lifestyle. The remaining two clan families, accounting for 30 per cent of the population, are the _Digil_ and _Rahanwayn_ clans, who originally followed an agricultural way of life.

The first refugees from Somalia came to the UK from the urban areas. Others followed later from the rural communities, their flights paid for by relatives already living in the UK, under a Home Office scheme that allowed residents to bring their families to the UK to join them.

Historically, Somalis have demonstrated an unwillingness to submit to authority and have a strong sense of independence. Despite sharing the same language, religion and customs, Somalis have developed a clear clan consciousness. This has led to conflict between different clans and sub-clans.

Religion

Somalis are generally Sunni Muslims.

Diet

Somalis do not eat pork or pork products. Any meat consumed must be _halal_, which is produced by slaughtering the animal in accordance with religious practices. Alcohol is forbidden.

Dress code

Somali men in the UK will generally wear western clothes, although they may also wear a white cloth cap. Somali women wear a scarf to cover their heads and a long gown known as a _juba_, which drapes from the neck to the ankles. This is because religious practice requires women to keep their bodies covered at all times.

Naming system

The Somali naming system differs from that of most Muslims. A Somali name is made up of the first/personal name with either the father's or grandfather's name used as a last name/surname. This naming system is used by both men and women. A typical male name is Personal Father Grandfather *Mohammed Jama Abdi*. A typical female name is *Sashra Omar Hassan*.

Women have traditionally maintained their own name on marriage and a husband and wife will often have names that have no common element.

Many Somalis had to leave their country in dangerous circumstances. To enable safe passage out of the country and avoid detection by rival clans, they had to use false names. These false names have subsequently appeared on their documentation in the host country and have by default become their legal names. However, members of their clan who are in their community in the host country are likely only to know them by the original name they had in Somalia.

Language

The predominant language of the Somali people is Somali. This had no written form until an official script was introduced in 1973. Because of this, many older people in the Somali community are unable to read and write, particularly those originating from the rural communities.

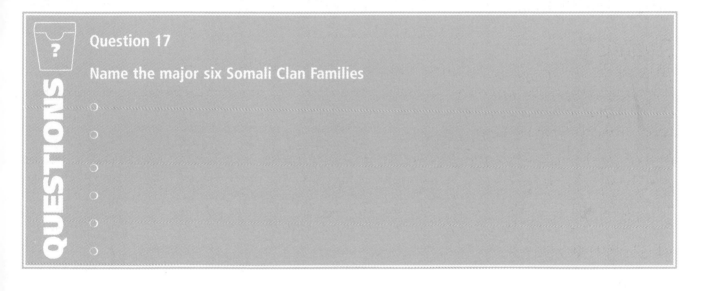

QUESTIONS

Question 17

Name the major six Somali Clan Families

○ ....

○ ....

○ ....

○ ....

○ ....

○ ....

Transgender people

There are believed to be around 500,000 transgender people in the UK. The precise number is not known. Many transgender people live without undergoing transition and live 'normal lives', either in their new gender or by changing from one gender to another depending on the situation. A large proportion of transgender people is to be found in London because of the existence of facilities such as specialist shops and a transgender community.

It is important to establish a few basic facts, as the myths and stereotypes surrounding transgender people are in most cases ill informed and incorrect.

Transgender people are uncomfortable in their birth gender. Some resolve this by undergoing re-assignment surgery, some live with the discomfort and conform to the roles expected of them by society, and others live with two identities – one for work and another in less formal situations. However a person deals with any discomfort with their gender, the issue is about identity not sexuality.

Terms and Definitions

○ *Biological sex*, being male or female as determined by chromosomes and body chemistry.

○ *Gender Expressed*, in terms of masculinity and femininity. It is how people present themselves and how they expect others to behave.

○ *Gender Identity*, the gender we identify with or feel that we belong to, i.e. male or female.

○ *Transvestism*, in the context of transgender people, the adoption, fully or partially, of the clothes normally identified as belonging to the opposite gender.

○ *Transsexuals*, profound form of gender dysphasia, in which individuals believe that they do not belong in the sex in which they were born and who have changed or are in the process of changing to their chosen sex or gender.

○ *Tran phobia*, animosity towards and/or irrational fear of transgender people.

○ *Tran phobic incident*, any incident that is perceived to be tran phobic by the victim or any other person. In effect, any incident intended to have an impact on those perceived to be transgender. As can be seen from the above definitions, the term 'sex' is referred to only in regards to biological sex. Few transvestites and transsexuals are gay. In fact only a small percentage of the transgender community self-identify as being lesbian, gay or bisexual. Very few people will fit neatly within one of these categories.

QUESTIONS

?

Question 18

Define the following words:

○ Transvestism

○ Transsexual

○ Tran phobic

_____

_____

Vietnamese

Most Vietnamese arrived in the UK in the late 1970s and throughout the 1980s. Many were forced to leave Vietnam as refugees to escape political and religious persecution. The Vietnamese community has originated from both North and South Vietnam and from rural and urban backgrounds. Its members originate from either ethnic Chinese or Vietnamese cultural backgrounds. The vast majority of Vietnamese immigrants are of ethnic Chinese descent. Although many adhere to Chinese customs, they consider themselves to be Vietnamese, as their families have been resident in North Vietnam for several generations. As a minority in Vietnam, accounting for less than 2 per cent of the population, many fled Vietnam after the 1978 war between China and Vietnam.

Religion

Most Vietnamese are either Buddhists or Catholics. Some also follow Chinese and Vietnamese customs of ancestor worship.

Diet

Vietnamese who are practising Buddhists may not eat meat. Those who are practising Catholics may not eat meat in Lent or on Fridays, when fish provides a suitable alternative.

Naming system

There are three parts to a Vietnamese name, with the family name coming first, followed by a complementary name and then personal name. In the UK, many Vietnamese anglicise their names by giving their family name last. It is unusual for a married woman to adopt her husband's family name.

Often, it is not possible to determine gender from an individual's personal name. However, complementary names can sometimes indicate sex: *Van* is often used by men and *This* by women as a complementary name.

Language

The predominant language of the Vietnamese is Vietnamese, although a few also speak Cantonese.

QUESTIONS

Question 19

a. What is the predominant language of the Vietnamese?

_____

_____

b. What religion do most Vietnamese follow?

_____

_____

Disability

This section is linked to DN16.1 and DN16.3.

This section of the handbook has been produced with the kind assistance of the Employers' Forum on Disability. It includes guidance on how to:

○ Assist people with specific impairments

○ Help develop a greater understanding of the views and preferences of disabled people in general

○ Recognise and avoid the attitudes and behaviour that could create barriers and misunderstandings.

The Race Relations (amended) Act 2000 places a new general statutory duty on public sector organisations to:

○ Eliminate unlawful discrimination

○ Promote equality of opportunity

○ Promote good race relations between people of different racial groups

37

☞

The Disability Discrimination Act 1999 makes it unlawful for service providers to treat disabled people less favourably for a reason related to their disability

QUESTIONS

Question 20

How Can We Promote People's Equality, Diversity and Rights in the Dental Environment?

Answer yes or no to the following statements to assess if your clients have equal access to your facilities.

a) Our surgery has a ramp over/next to the front steps, but the hygienist has a surgery on the first floor and we do not have a lift

b) Emergency patients are seen on a first come first served basis

c) The female toilet on the ground floor is very small

d) The waiting area has beautiful soft sofas

e) The Dentist usually runs 20–30mins late

If you have answered yes to any of the above you may unwittingly be discriminating against your patients

For each of the above statements, list reasons why you may be seen to be discriminating against your patients.

Suggestions

○ If a client is in a wheelchair or pushing a child in a pram, they may be able to gain access to the building, but not to see the hygienist (a)

○ First come first served (b) may not take into account parents who have to take young children to school or people who have to eat at regular intervals, for example diabetics.

○ Small toilets (c) do not assist clients in wheelchairs or people with young children in buggies.

○ Soft sofas (d) may be very attractive but if a person has arthritis or has had knee/hip replacements they need firm arms on the chair to help them push upwards out of the seat.

○ Running 20–30mins late (e) discriminates against people who have to collect children from school or people who need to take regular medication.

Think again

What can we do to ensure that we treat people equally?

QUESTIONS

Question 21

List 5 improvements that could be made to your work environment

○

○

○

○

○

Language

The language that we use and the way that we use it can either be a vehicle for our prejudices, or a way of showing that we care about giving fair treatment. For example, it is insensitive to refer to a person who has arthritis as 'arthritic' or a person who has cerebral palsy as 'spastic'. They are PEOPLE who have a condition that disables them.

QUESTIONS

Question 22

Complete the last line:

○ Invalid   –   wheelchair user

○ Victim of   –   person who has/people with

○ Mental handicap   –

Disability affects one in four people

Disability is not always immediately obvious. There may be no visible signs, such as a white stick or crutches. Fewer than 5 per cent of disabled people, around 400,000, use a wheelchair all the time.

❍ There are 8.7 million disabled people in the UK.

❍ 5.5 million are of working age.

❍ One in four adults is disabled or close to someone who is.

The changing climate

The position of disabled people in society is changing. With improved technology and a better understanding of disability, a greater number of disabled people can enjoy a full life; they can follow careers that are appropriate to their talents, and use services and buildings that are gradually becoming accessible to everyone.

Communication

As you think about the best way to work with and to serve people with disabilities, communication is probably the first thing that comes to mind. Using language sensitively and having good communication skills make it easier to treat everyone as you yourself would expect to be treated. You will understand that certain language and behaviour can cause offence. There can be misunderstandings, perhaps because you think of disability in terms of dated stereotypes or simply because you may have had very little personal contact with disabled people. This lack of understanding can create unnecessary barriers and can even result in discrimination.

Watch, ask and listen

Perhaps you want to improve your communication with disabled people. Although the important thing is always to ask, and to take your lead from the person, this section will give you some basics to build on through your own contact with disabled people. Remember to keep in touch with what individuals prefer.

Communication skills can go a very long way. Watch carefully, really listen to people, and only then offer help and adjustments. This is vital to treating someone with respect and consideration – whether or not they seem to be disabled. Be alert to the needs of others.

The Disability Discrimination Act (1995) (DDA)

The Disability Discrimination Act (1995) (DDA) protects people with a wide range of impairments – for example, dyslexia, epilepsy, severe facial disfigurement, angina, ME and mental health problems. The parts of the Act that relate to employment apply to every organisation with 15 or more employees. More measures to protect disabled customers are being introduced between October 1999 and January 2004. The customer-related responsibilities apply to all organisations, however small.

Some basics

Removing barriers is not just about spending money on structural alterations. 'Access' should be applied in its broadest sense, to all communications and opportunities.

The Act protects individuals who have, or have ever had, any mental or physical impairment that lasted, or is expected to last, at least 12 months, and which has a substantial adverse effect on their day-to-day activities.

Disability is not sickness – the general health of most disabled people is as good as that of anyone else. When meeting a disabled person:

❍   Only offer help if it seems appropriate. Always wait until your offer is accepted before you do anything; listen to what the person says.

❍   Only use a disabled person's first name if you are also using other people's first names.

❍   Treat a disabled person with the same respect you would give to anyone else.

❍   Do not treat disabled adults as children.

❍   Do not lean on someone's wheelchair: it is his or her personal space.

❍   Communicate directly with the disabled person, not to their companion or interpreter.

❍   Only make the same physical contact as you would make with anyone else; do not help someone to get up or sit down without first offering to help and listening to his or her reply.

❍   Do not use extravagant gestures or language that draws attention to the person's disability.

Language

Certain words and phrases may give offence. Although there are no hard and fast rules, it is helpful to understand the background.

Some people prefer to be called 'disabled people', which they believe gives the message that they are disabled by society's barriers. Others prefer to be called 'people with disabilities', which they believe gives the message that they are people first, who also have a disability. Preferences change with time. Ask people what they prefer. Do not be embarrassed about using common expressions that could relate to someone's impairment, for example 'see you later' or 'I'll be running along then'. Many people object to the word 'handicapped', which has been used by many charities over the years, as they believe it reinforces the message that disabled people are dependent on charity.

People do not want to be given a medical label, which can be very misleading: no two people are the same. Labels say little about the individual, they just reinforce stereotypes of disabled people as being 'sick' and dependent on the medical profession.

○ You should say 'someone with cerebral palsy' and never 'a spastic'; and 'someone with epilepsy' and not 'an epileptic'.

○ The phrase 'mental handicap' has been replaced by 'people with learning disabilities'. People with learning disabilities are increasingly speaking for themselves and this is their preference.

○ You should not use collective nouns such as 'the disabled', 'the blind', 'the deaf', 'the disfigured'; these terms imply that people are part of a uniform group that is separate from the rest of society.

○ You should never use insulting labels like 'cripple', 'retarded', 'blind as a bat' or 'mentally defective' even as a joke, whether or not a disabled person is present.

○ Do not use language that suggests disabled people are always frail or dependent on others, or which could make disabled people objects of pity. Also, you should remember that the opposite of 'disabled' is not 'able-bodied'. This suggests that disability is only physical. Non-disabled means 'neither physically nor mentally disabled'.

Meeting people with impaired vision

○ Introduce yourself and other people clearly; say where people are in the room.

○ A guide dog is a working dog and should not be treated as a pet.

○ If the person seems to need help, ask 'may I offer you an arm?'; that way, you can guide rather than seeming to propel the person.

○ When you are offering a handshake say 'shall we shake hands?'.

○ When you are offering a seat, guide the person's hand to the back or the arm of the seat, and say that is what you are going to do.

○ Offer minutes of meetings or any other written communications in the person's preferred format (on floppy disk, in large print, on audio cassette or in Braille).

○ Where someone might normally take notes, ask if they would like to tape the meeting or conversation.

○ Tell the person if you are going to move away, so that they are not left talking into empty space.

Meeting people who are deaf

○ There are different degrees and types of deafness, and different ways for deaf people or those who are hard of hearing to communicate.

○ Ask the person to tell you how they prefer to communicate, and to help you to find and book interpreters or other support in advance.

○ If there is a sign language interpreter, speak to the individual not to the interpreter.

○ You might also need lip-speakers (trained to speak in a way that lip-readers will find easy to understand) or palantype operators (speed-text communicators, using laptops or a larger screen) to help you to communicate.

○ Look directly at the person you are speaking to; stop talking if you have to turn away.

○ Speak clearly in normal speech rhythm and a little more slowly.

○ Do not use exaggerated gestures.

○ Make sure you are visible in a good light.

○ Do not block your mouth with your hands, cigarettes or food (very important to remember this in a medical / dental setting when masks are worn).

Meeting people who are deaf-blind

Deaf-blindness is a combination of hearing and sight impairments, but deaf-blind people are not always completely deaf and blind. In fact, most deaf-blind people do have some residual hearing or sight, or both. So, the advice provided in the sections on people with impaired vision or hearing may also apply. In addition:

○ Let the person know you are there: approach from the front and touch them lightly on the arm or shoulder to attract their attention.

○ Many deaf-blind people need to be guided. Different people like to be guided in different ways: some deaf-blind people experience poor balance.

○ Do not grab or propel or pull a person – let them know you are offering to escort them by guiding their hand to your elbow.

○ Communication methods used by deaf-blind people can include the following:– lip-reading;– writing notes;– sign language, which a specially skilled interpreter might adapt for the person;– block alphabet: this is where you use your forefinger to write words on the palm of the deaf-blind person's hand – use the whole palm and write in clear capital letters;– deaf-blind manual alphabet.

Meeting people who use a wheelchair or crutches

○ If you are talking for more than a few moments to someone in a wheelchair, try to position yourself so that you are at the same level, or at least ask the person if they would like you to sit down.

○ If there is a high desk or counter, move to the front.

○ Do not tidy away someone's crutches when they sit down.

○ If you know it is not easy to move around your building in a wheelchair, offer to help: heavy doors or deep-pile carpets are just some of the hazards to watch for.

○ Do not assume that ramps solve everything – they may be too steep or too slippery.

Meeting people with speech difficulties

○ Pay attention to a person with speech difficulties; be patient and be encouraging – do not butt in and finish sentences.

○ Slowness or impaired speech has nothing to do with someone's intelligence. If you need information, break down your questions to deal with individual points.

○ Do not pretend to understand if you have not.

Meeting people with mental health problems

People with a past history of mental health problems can experience discrimination. Most people make a full recovery. However, someone experiencing the emotional distress and confusion associated with mental health problems may find everyday activities difficult. Be patient and non-judgemental. Give the person time to make decisions.

Meeting people with learning disabilities

Many people born with learning disabilities, and people in the early stages of dementia or who acquire a brain injury, live full and independent lives in the community, making their own choices, with varying levels of support. These notes may apply to any of these individuals.

○ Start by assuming that the person will understand you; be prepared to explain things more than once in different ways.

○ Break down complicated information to give one piece at a time: preview and review it.

○ Keep distractions (background noise and bustle) to a minimum.

○ Consider putting information in writing, including your name and phone number; perhaps offer to tape a conversation so that the person can consider it later and keep a record.

Meeting people with facial disfigurement

Some people are born with a disfigurement and others acquire it through an accident or illness. Disfigurement is 'only skin-deep'. Like any disability, it does not mean the person is any different and certainly does not affect his or her intelligence. Most of the difficulties, indeed discrimination, people with facial disfigurement experience, stem from other people's behaviour.

○ If you are surprised by someone's appearance, or feel uncomfortable, try not to show it.

○ Make eye contact, as you would with anyone else; try not to stare.

○ Listen carefully, and do not let the person's appearance distract you.

○ Never ask 'what happened to you?' Restrain your curiosity.

QUESTIONS

?

Question 23

List the three communication methods that can be used by blind-deaf people.

○

○

○

Terminology

This section contains guidance on appropriate terminology in relation to key groups and communities. It is intended as a general guide and is not exhaustive. Also, terminology changes constantly. The general rule is that if you are unsure about what term or expression to use you should always ask the individual how they would prefer to be addressed. This can be used in conjunction with the 'key words' from DN16.1, DN16.2 and DN16.3.

Ethnic minorities

The term 'ethnic minority' is most frequently used to describe people who share a common sense of identity based on shared kinship, culture, language, religion, history or country of origin. It is recognised, however, that some people will feel that this term does not adequately describe their origins, background or identity.

In some cases, the expression 'minority ethnic' is also used. This tends to be used in a collective context – as in 'minority ethnic communities' rather than in the singular. An individual would be unlikely to say, for example, 'I am a minority ethnic'.

The term 'minority ethnic' also seeks to acknowledge that it is not just the 'minority' but also the 'majority' that has an ethnic identity.

The term 'ethnics' should be avoided. The Commission for Racial Equality and the British National Census Office recommended the following ethnic origin categories for use in the 2001 Census.

It is likely that these will be adopted by most public bodies and organisations to enable data comparison.

1. White: (i) British (ii) Irish (iii) Other

2. Mixed: (i) White and Black Caribbean (ii) White and Black African (iii) White and Asian

3. Asian or Asian British: (i) Indian (ii) Pakistani (iii) Bangladeshi (iv) Any other Asian background

4. Black or Black British: (i) Caribbean (ii) African (iii) Any other Black background

5. Chinese or other ethnic group: (i) Chinese (ii) Any other

Terms relating to skin colour

KEY WORDS

Black, it is generally acceptable to use the term 'Black' to describe members of the Black-African, African-Caribbean and Black-British communities. This is how members of these communities often describe themselves, as in Black Association, Black Churches or Black Music. In some cases, the term is applied generically to other 'visible' minorities, for example to members of the Asian community. It should be noted, however, that many Asians do not describe themselves in this way. Some people who are not of African origin choose to describe themselves as Black. This is often a political definition designed to express solidarity with others subjected to racism.

Coloured, it is not appropriate to use the term 'coloured'. The term has many negative connotations, including its association with South African apartheid and the UK in the 1950s and 1960s when signs stating 'uncoloured' were commonly displayed in shops, public houses and hotels. The expression 'people of colour' is commonly used in the United States but it is probably best avoided in a British context as it is not a common term. It may be misunderstood or misinterpreted by some people.

Half-caste, it is not acceptable to use the term 'half-caste', which has been used to describe people whose parents are from different ethnic, cultural or racial groups. A preferred term is 'mixed race', although this too will not be acceptable to all groups. The 2001 Census categories included the following ethnic origin classifications: Mixed – White and Black Caribbean; Mixed – White and Asian; Mixed – Any other mixed background. Another term is '*bi-cultural*'.

Specific ethnic groups

KEY WORDS

Afro-Caribbean/African-Caribbean Has traditionally been used to describe people who are historically of African origin but who have migrated to the UK from the Caribbean Islands. Some people prefer to be called African-Caribbean or Black-British because they feel that this more accurately reflects their experience and identity. The term '*West Indian*' is no longer in common use, although some people may describe themselves in this way.

African The term 'African' is acceptable and is often used in self-identification. Many people, however, will refer to themselves in national terms, as in Nigerian, Ghanaian, etc.

Asian It is acceptable to use the expression 'Asian', which generally relates to people originating from the Indian sub-continent (South Asia) Indians, Pakistanis and Bangladeshis (although Asia extends from Turkey to China). Many members of these communities will not identify as Asian, however, preferring to describe themselves in relation to their particular racial, cultural or national origin.

Chinese It is acceptable to use the term 'Chinese'. The term 'oriental' should be avoided.

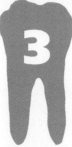

3 MEDICAL EMERGENCIES

This chapter is linked to DN01.3 of the NVQ Level 3 in Oral Health Care.

Medical emergencies can happen within the dental surgery and this chapter looks at:

○ Emergency drugs and equipment

○ Patient monitoring

○ Medical emergency management

○ First aid.

Professional Conduct and Fitness to Practise/General Dental Council (Paragraph 27)

A patient could collapse in the dental surgery at any time and the collapse may not be associated with the dental treatment or with the administration of general anaesthesia or sedation. Dentists should therefore ensure that all members of their staff are properly trained and prepared to deal with an emergency should one arise. The requirement to practise resuscitation routines frequently in a simulated emergency against the clock is not restricted to that dentist who practices sedation in their surgeries. The council also considers it essential that suction apparatus to clear the oropharynx, oral airways to maintain a natural airway; equipment with appropriate attachments to provide intermittent positive pressure to the lungs; and a portable source of oxygen with administration attachments must be available in all dental practices. In this connection, the current guidelines issued by the European Resuscitation Council should be adopted.
May 1996

Paying close attention to the importance of complete medical histories for patients, which should be updated every six months and confirmed that no changes have taken place on each visit to the surgery, can help to prevent emergencies. However, as the above paragraph states, emergencies do happen and the dental team should be fully prepared to manage the situation.

Emergency drugs and equipment

Drugs

It is recommended that the following drugs should be held within the dental practice (the list is documented in the Dental Practitioner Formulary along with administration advice):

○ Salbutamol inhaler

○ Salbutamol for IV injection (500mcgs/ml; 1ml amp)

○ Adrenaline Epine phrine 1.1000 (1mg/ml for intra muscular (IM); 3 x 1ml amps)

○ Aspirin dispersible tablets (300mg)

○ Chlorphenamine injection (10mg/ml; 3 x 1ml amps)

○ Diazepam injection (5mg /ml; 3 x 2ml amps)

- ○ Glucagon injection (I unit vial with solvent)

- ○ Glucose powder

- ○ Glucose intravenous infusion 50% (1 x 50ml pre-filled syringe)

- ○ Glyceryl trinitrate tablets or sprays

- ○ Hydrocortisone injection (100mg vial + 2ml sterile water for injection)

- ○ Oxygen

The drugs should be secured when the surgery is not in use, but readily available during the working day – when you have an emergency you do not want to go hunting for the key! A record should be kept of the drugs and the expiry dates noted and checked. Located with the drugs should be the necessary equipment required to administer the drugs, for example, syringes/hypodermic needles/alcohol swabs/labels.

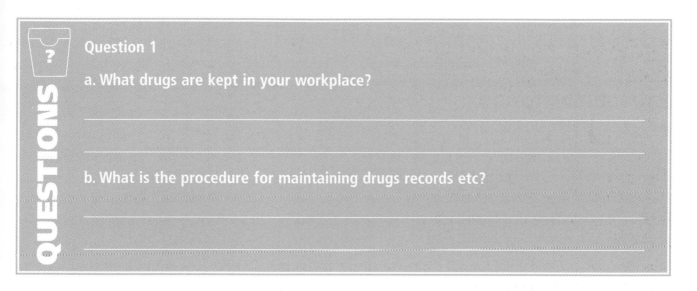

QUESTIONS

? **Question 1**

a. What drugs are kept in your workplace?

_____

_____

b. What is the procedure for maintaining drugs records etc?

_____

_____

Emergency equipment

To support breathing and ventilation, the equipment recommended to be held within the surgery is:

- ○ Bag valve and mask with reservoir

- ○ Pocket face mask

- ○ Oropharyngeal airways

- ○ Nasal airways

- ○ Portable suction and tubing

- ○ Independent hand-operated suction

- ○ Portable oxygen, mask and tubing

As with the emergency drugs, the above equipment should be checked regularly for functionality and a record kept of the checks made. Oxygen cylinder valves sometime stick or, if the oxygen has been left flowing, the cylinder may have emptied – the time to discover this is not when you need it in an emergency. Regular checks, either daily or weekly, should be carried out routinely.

Question 2

a. Where does your surgery keep their emergency equipment?

_____

b. Is the equipment checked daily or weekly?

_____

c. Create a chart for keeping the checks recorded

_____

d. Why is it important to do these regular checks?

_____

Patient monitoring

A 'monitor' is a person or an object that gives a warning or reminder.

It is important to monitor each patient from the time they enter the practice, even when they are in the waiting room – dental treatment can be very stressful for many patients and emergencies can happen in the waiting room as well as the surgery.

The dental nurse (DN) can act as an important monitor, and one who can care for the patient throughout their dental procedure and report any changes or concerns to the dentist. In the reception/waiting room area this responsibility usually rests upon the receptionist, which is why it is important for all members of the team to attend regular emergency training sessions.

Patient monitoring involves the observation of physiological parameters over a period of time in order to detect any changes and deal with them before a potentially dangerous situation develops. This is done by observation of:

❍ General appearance of the patient (e.g. sweating, shaking, nervous mannerism)

❍ Level of consciousness (e.g. are they fully responsive?)

❍ Muscle tone (e.g. tense or staggering and unable to walk)

❍ Colour of skin and mucosa (e.g. sudden pallor)

❍ Respiratory pattern (e.g. too fast or too slow; very noisy).

☞ See section on emergency diagnosis.

A DN should be able to locate and record a patient's pulse when necessary. Usually the radial pulse is the pulse of choice, which is located at the wrist where the artery passes across the radius bone. The pulse is best felt by using the forefinger and middle finger, placing them approximately $1/2 - 1$ inch from the junction of the arm to hand; gentle pressure applied will locate the artery, the forefinger measuring the rate of the pulse beats and the middle finger judging the strength. Time the pulse beats using the second hand of a clock or watch, counting the beats for $1/2$ a minute and then times by two, this will give the pulse rate per minute.

QUESTIONS

Question 3

Take and record the pulse rate of your colleagues. How would you expect the pulse rate to be affected by anxiety and why?

_____

_____

_____

_____

For the majority of patients undergoing treatment with local anaesthesia this level of monitoring is sufficient, however, additional monitoring is required if the patient is undergoing sedation.

See chapter on Conscious Sedation.

QUESTIONS

Question 4

Write a reflective account on three patients undergoing dental treatment whom you have monitored. How did any nervousness show, e.g. colour of complexion etc.?

_____

_____

_____

_____

Medical emergency management and first aid

Burns

It is important to assess a burn before treatment commences. You need to look at the circumstances that caused the injury, the type, extent, location and depth of the burn.

The main types of burn risk within the dental environment are:

○ Heat/flame (Autoclave/hot air burner/bunsen burner)

○ Liquid/steam (Autoclave/kettle)

○ Scald/liquid (Autoclave/kettle/tea/coffee)

○ Cold injury (Ethyl chloride)

○ Chemical burns (Sodium hypochlorite/sterilising solution/acid etch)

○ Electrical burns (Using any electrical equipment if the flexes or plugs are faulty)

The extent of the burn will indicate if the patient is at risk from shock (referred to later on). Shock is a life-threatening situation and occurs whenever there is a major loss of body fluid; in severe extensive burns fluid loss is largely due to the body fluid serum (colourless fluid) leaking through the damaged skin and sometimes forming blisters. Burns also allow bacteria to enter the skin and the risk of infection is high.

Minor burns

○ Cool the affected area immediately with cold water and continue for at least ten minutes to stop the burning and pain.

○ Put on clean gloves and remove any jewellery or clothing that may become constrictive if the damaged area swells.

○ Cover the area with clean and sterile dressing. Do not puncture any blisters that may develop.

Although most minor burns can be dealt with by the above procedure, if at all concerned, medical advice should be sought.

Severe burns

○ Lay the patient down.

○ Dial 999 for an ambulance.

○ Cool the injured area with water for at least ten minutes.

○ Put on clean gloves and remove any jewellery or clothing that may become constrictive if the affected area swells.

○ Carefully remove any burnt clothing, unless it is sticking to the wound. DO NOT ATTEMPT TO REMOVE CLOTHING THAT IS STICKING TO THE WOUND.

○ Cover the injured area with sterile dressing or, if the area is too large, a sheet of cling film applied lengthways. A clean plastic bag can also be used for hands and feet.

○ Monitor the patient and treat for shock (referred to later on).

☞

When cooling the affected area, especially if the area is extensive, care should be taken not to overcool the body, because this is hazardous in the elderly and babies.

Do not remove any clothing sticking to wound.

Do not puncture blisters.

Do not apply creams or ointment.

Do not touch the burnt area.

Question 5

Why should the DN remove gloves when using a bunsen burner or any heat source, e.g. sealing gutta percha?

_____

_____

_____

_____

Eye injury

The most common eye injuries are caused by small flecks of dust or a loose eyelash that can float on the white of the eye – usually such objects can be rinsed off. However, you must not touch anything that sticks to, penetrates or rests on the iris or pupil as this can damage the eye. Medical assistance should be sought immediately.

Should chemical substances splash into the eye, reference should be immediately made to the COSHH sheet (see DN01) for that substance and treatment carried out as advised.

Foreign object in the eye

- Advise the patient to sit down facing the light.

- Tell them not to rub the eye.

- Stand behind the patient.

- Gently separate the eyelids with your finger and thumb.

- Examine every part of the eye.

- If you can see a foreign object on the white of the eye wash it out by pouring clean water from a glass or by using a sterile eyewash.

- If this is unsuccessful, lift the object off with a moist swab or the damp corner of a clean handkerchief or tissue.

- If you still cannot remove the object seek medical advice.

Poisons

Chemicals that are swallowed may not only harm the digestive tract and invade the blood system, affecting other parts of the body including breathing and circulation, but can also cause severe burning and swelling within the throat, creating a risk to breathing.

The COSHH folder held within each dental practice should contain the data information for each chemical substance. Within this data will be the emergency guidelines to be followed in the event of misuse through inhalation, ingestion (swallowing), skin contact or eye contact. This data sheet should be consulted prior to treatment commencing as the treatment can differ with different substances.

○ If the patient is conscious ask them what they have swallowed and reassure.

○ Dial 999 for an ambulance; give as much information as possible about the swallowed poison.

☞ Do not induce vomiting

○ If the patient becomes unconscious open the airway and check breathing; be prepared to give rescue breathing and basic life support.

○ If the patient loses consciousness but is breathing, place into the recovery position and constantly monitor breathing and pulse.

○ If the patient has swallowed chemicals use a face shield, pocket face mask or ventilating bag, in case there are chemicals still on the patient's mouth.

QUESTIONS

Question 5

a. Where is the COSHH data kept in your surgery and is it up to date?

_____

_____

b. Read through the data and learn the emergency guidelines for the substances used in your surgery

_____

_____

Fractures

A fracture is a break or crack in the bone. Fractures can occur in several ways, through direct force, such as being hit by a car, and indirect force, such as a twist or a wrench. The signs of a fracture injury may be:

○ Deformity

○ Swelling

○ Pain

○ Twisting or bending of limb

○ Grating when moved

○ Wound with bone ends penetrating.

If you suspect a fracture:

○ Keep the patient still.

○ Support the injured area until immobilised.

○ Immobilise the injured area by bandaging it to an unaffected area of the body, e.g. support an injured leg by bandaging it to the uninjured leg.

❍ Arrange transport to hospital immediately.

❍ Treat for shock (see section later in chapter).

❍ Check circulation beyond the bandage every ten minutes; if the circulation is impaired, loosen the bandage.

❍ Do not attempt to straighten limbs as this may cause internal damage to major blood vessels and nerves.

❍ Do not move the patient until the injured part is secured and supported.

❍ Do not give anything to eat or drink, as an anaesthetic may be needed.

☞ If there is an open wound put on clean gloves and cover the injured area with a large, sterile dressing. Do not press down on the protruding bone.

Bleeding wounds

When a blood vessel is damaged, several mechanisms click into action within the body to overcome the injury and prevent blood loss, by forming a blood clot. However, in extensive wounds or wounds to major blood vessels, uncontrolled blood loss can occur before these mechanisms can take place. Severe blood loss will lead to shock (referred to later on).

There are various types of wounds depending on how the injury was caused, e.g. stab wound/abrasion/gunshot/puncture/contusion.

☞ The aim is to control bleeding, prevent shock, minimise infection and seek medical attention.

No object in wound

❍ With gloves on, apply direct pressure over the wound with your fingers or palm, preferably over a clean dressing pad.

❍ Raise or elevate the injured limb above the heart level to reduce bleeding.

❍ Lie the patient down and keep warm to prevent shock.

❍ Secure the dressing with a bandage that is tight enough to maintain pressure, but not so tight that it restricts circulation.

❍ If further bleeding occurs apply a second dressing on top of the first.

❍ If blood soaks through this, remove both dressings and apply fresh dressings, ensuring that the pressure point is accurate to point of bleeding.

❍ Support injured limb.

❍ Dial 999 and transfer to hospital.

Object in wound

❍ As above but **do not press the object into wound** when controlling bleeding.

❍ Place dressing either side of the object, building up on each side until able to bandage without pressure on the object.

Cuts and grazes

❍ Wear gloves and wash the wound under running water.

❍ Pat wound dry gently with gauze swab.

❍ Cover with sterile dressing.

❍ Elevate the limb where possible.

- ○ Clean surrounding areas.

- ○ Pat dry.

- ○ Remove wound dressing and apply a fresh dressing.

- ○ If unable to clean wound thoroughly seek medical advice.

QUESTIONS

? Question 6

Who is the first aider in your workplace?

A comprehensive first aid manual should be located with the first aid box for reference. A recommended course for DNs to attend is the 'First Aider in the Workplace'. This provides the DN with up-to-date practical skills and carries with it a three-year certificate.

☞ Recommended reading 'DK First Aid Manual', the authorised manual of the St John's Ambulance, St Andrew's Ambulance Ass, and the British Red Cross.

First aid box

This box should be **green with a white cross** and recommended contents are:

- ○ Disposable gloves

- ○ Face mask

- ○ Six safety pins

- ○ Gauze pads

- ○ 20 adhesive dressings ass*

- ○ Six medium sterile dressings

- ○ Two large sterile dressings

- ○ Two extra-large sterile dressings

- ○ Two sterile eye pads*

- ○ Six triangular bandages

- ○ Two crepe roller bandages

- Scissors
- Tweezers
- Cotton wool
- Non-alcoholic wound cleansing wipes
- Adhesive tapes**
- Notepad and pencil

* It is recommended that a bottle of sterile eye wash solution is kept with the first aid box

** Certain protocols within your own workplace may influence the use of adhesive plasters and tape

Question 7

a. Where is your first aid box located and are the contents up to date?

b. Why is it important to record all accidents and what information should be included in the record?

Medical emergency in the dental surgery

The fear, anxiety and stress that some people experience with dental treatment can have an effect on the respiratory and cardio-vascular system, and may exacerbate any predisposing illness or disease. It is therefore essential that the dental team and the dental surgery are thoroughly prepared to cope with an emergency should it arise. The dental team should be capable in the management of medical emergencies and fully competent in the provision of basic life support and the use of resuscitation equipment.

Airway management

Patients requiring resuscitation often have obstructed airways, either as the cause or effect of loss of consciousness. Quick assessment and immediate action in the establishment of a patent airway is of paramount importance if cerebral hypoxic damage is to be avoided.

Airway obstruction can be caused by many factors, and can be complete or partial, affecting either the upper or lower respiratory tract or both. Upper respiratory obstruction may be occlusion of the oropharynx, hypopharynx and nasopharynx by either the tongue, epiglottis, soft palate or other soft tissue and this is most common in unconscious patients. Blood, vomit and foreign material can also obstruct the upper airway. Laryngeal obstruction can be caused by swelling (oedema), spasm (caused by fumes or irritants) or a foreign object.

Lower airway obstruction can be caused by:

○ Brachial secretions

○ Mucus plug obstructing bronchi

○ Pulmonary haemorrhage

○ Pneumothorax (following trauma to lung)

○ Pulmonary oedema (swelling obstructing lung function)

○ Aspiration of vomit.

Recognition of airway obstruction

LOOK – Chest Movement

  – Abdominal Movement

LISTEN – Sounds of airflow

FEEL – Movement of airflow

In partial airway obstruction, movement of the chest and abdomen is greatly exaggerated, and inspiratory noises are noticeable, crowing and snoring are also detectable. Obstruction of the lower airway usually presents as a wheeze. Gurgling could indicate presence of liquid or a semi-solid material.

Opening the airway

Once obstruction has been recognised immediate action should be taken to correct the situation and maintain a clear airway. Following the correct method of opening the airway, 'head tilt; chin lift' should result in relieving airway obstruction where relaxed soft tissues are the cause. When this is not successful other causes of obstruction must be sought and remedied. Any obvious foreign material in the mouth, such as a displaced denture, should also be removed. Well-fitting dentures should be left in place as they help to maintain a mouth seal during ventilation.

Head tilt; chin lift

The airway in patients can be occluded by the base of the tongue and the breathing obstructed as a result. An oropharyngeal airway (guedal) may not be enough to prevent obstruction, since these can become blocked with secretions. Failure to maintain an unobstructed airway in the unconscious patient may be overcome by the simple manoeuvre of head tilt; by stretching the anterior neck muscles, the base of the tongue is lifted from the posterior pharyngeal wall and the epiglottis from the laryngeal inlet. Further stretching of these muscles is produced by lifting the chin, to pull the mandible and thus also the tongue forward.

○ If possible support the head on a small cushion.

○ Extend the head on the neck by pushing the forehead backwards and the occiput posteriorly.

○ Simultaneously place two fingers under the tip of the mandible and lift the chin, displacing the tongue forward.

○ If a neck injury is suspected, do not tilt the head unless other methods of opening the airway have failed. Reduce the risk of further injury by minimising neck movements, but remember: **death from hypoxia caused by airway obstruction is more common than quadriplegia arising as a result of emergency airway manipulation**.

Jaw thrust

Jaw thrust is an additional manoeuvre that can relieve obstruction by the tongue, and is recommended when cervical injury is a possibility.

○ Hold the mouth slightly open by downward displacement of the chin with the thumbs.

○ With the index and other fingers, apply steady upward and forward pressure at the angles of the mandible to lift the jaw forward.

Mouth to mask ventilation

Simple ventilation adjuncts are available for use in expired air ventilation, which avoid direct person-to-person contact, therefore making the procedure more acceptable, especially when vomit and blood are present. In the dental area, where blood in the mouth is present in a high percentage of treatment cases, these appliances are recommended. These appliances can also reduce the risk of cross infection. Certain airways allow enrichment of oxygen to be delivered.

Pocket face mask

Pocket face masks also contain one-way valve ports, preventing contamination with body fluids.

○ Place the patient in the supine position (on their back) with airway aligned and, if possible, head supported on a small pillow.

○ Apply the mask to the patient's face with both hands by pressing with the thumbs and forefingers along the cushion edge of the mask.

○ Lift the jaw into the mask by exerting pressure with the remaining fingers of both hands at angles of the jaw to ensure a tight seal. Leaks can be abolished by adjusting fingers and hand pressure, or altering the jaw thrust.

○ If the mask has an oxygen port, add oxygen at 8–10 litres per minute, or the manufacturer's recommended rate.

○ Inflate the patient's lungs with expired air through the one-way mask valve port.

Pharyngeal airways

Oropharyngeal and nasopharyngeal airways are often helpful and sometimes essential in maintaining a patent airway, especially when the resuscitation is prolonged. The airway must still be aligned with head tilt and chin lift or jaw thrust, but the pharyngeal airways help to overcome tongue displacement. In the dental area, the situation could arise where the patient has extensive bleeding in the mouth causing further risk to the airway. The use of the nasopharyngeal airway is ideally suited in these cases as it enables oral bleeding to be arrested with packs, therefore preventing blood from being aspired into the lungs with each ventilation.

Oropharyngeal airway

Oropharyngeal airways (guedal) are curved plastic tubes reinforced at the oral end. They are available in sizes to suit the neonate through to large adult (00–5). The average adult female is size 3 and male adult size 4. An estimate of the size of airway required can be achieved by selecting an airway with a length corresponding to the distance between the corner of the mouth and the angle of the mandible.

During insertion of the airway care must be taken not to push the tongue or any debris further back into the pharynx, thus worsening not improving the airway. If laryngeal reflexes are present, vomiting or laryngospasm may occur and insertion should only take place in comatose patients.

○ Introduce the airway into the oral cavity in the inverted position and rotate it through 180 degrees as it passes below the palate and into the oropharynx. Incorrect insertion can push the tongue back and obstruct the airway.

○ If there is any retching, indicating laryngeal reflexes are present, the airway should be removed to avoid the risk of aspiration.

○ After insertion, check the patency and maintain correct alignment of the head and neck with chin lift or jaw thrust.

Nasopharyngeal airway

These tubes are generally tolerated better than the oropharyngeal, but their insertion can cause epistaxis (nose bleed). The use of soft tubes, lubrication and correct insertion can reduce this problem. Nasopharyngeal tubes must not be used if there is any suspicion of base of skull fracture, or signs of cerebral damage indicated by blood or clear fluid from ears or nose. A 6mm tube is usually selected for a woman and 7mm for a man.

○ Lubricate tube thoroughly.

○ Introduce the tube into the right nostril (the right nostril is usually the one of choice, if a person has a deviated septum it more often deviates to the left) and gently pass it directly backwards through the nasal cavity, so that the distal end lies in the hypopharynx.

○ If obstruction is met, do not force the tube, remove, and try the left nostril.

☞ **Nasopharanygeal tubes should never be inserted if there is indication of a fracture to the base of the skull.**

Ventilating by a self-inflating bag and valve

A self-inflating bag and valve allows a patient to be ventilated by either mask or tracheal tube, with the use of room air, oxygen-enriched air or pure oxygen. The bag on its own will impart approximately 20 per cent oxygen, however, with a reservoir bag connected to oxygen flow at 10 litres it can produce an inspirational value of 90 per cent+ oxygen. Without the reservoir bag, but with oxygen flowing at 6–8 litres into the self-inflating bag, it will produce an inspirational oxygen value of 50 per cent.

Manual compression of the bag inflates the lungs through an unidirectional valve; when the bag is released the patient's passive exhalation is diverted through the valve to the atmosphere and the bag fills with room air through the separate inlet valve.

Use of the self-inflating bag can achieve far higher oxygen concentration levels than mask and expired air, but it requires greater skill and it is often difficult to achieve a perfect seal between face and mask.

Method

○ Place the patient in a supine position with the airway aligned.

○ Apply the face mask and make an airtight seal. Encircle the circumference of the mask with the thumb and forefinger close to the patient valve connection. Apply upward jaw thrust with the little, ring and middle fingers to keep the face in contact with the mask.

○ Compress the bag to inflate the patient's lungs. Success is indicated by the rise and fall of the chest.

○ Excessive compression of the bag can lead to over-inflation, which results in gastric inflation, eventually leading to the risk of aspiration of stomach contents if the airway is less than perfectly patent. Cricoid pressure can reduce this risk but this requires the presence of a suitably trained assistant.

○ If a spare person is available, the bag can be compressed by the second person using two hands, and the mask held by the first person, again using both hands.

Basic life support

Guidelines are continually being updated so check with the latest Resuscitation Council Guidelines. Basic life support comprises the following elements:

○ Initial assessment + airway maintenance

○ Expired air ventilation

○ Cardiac compressions

The three combined constitute, Cardio Pulmonary Resuscitation (CPR). If a simple airway or face mask is used to aid ventilation, it is defined as basic life support with airway adjunct.

The purpose of basic life support is to maintain adequate ventilation and circulation to support life until the means can be obtained to reverse the underlying cause of the arrest. Basic life support is therefore a 'holding' procedure. Sometimes, however, when the underlying cause is purely respiratory, it may itself evoke full recovery. Failure of the circulation for upwards of three minutes will lead to irreversible cerebral damage (other than in rare hypothermic cases, e.g. immersion in cold water, where the sudden drop in body temperature lowers the amount of oxygen required by the body tissues). Delay in commencing basic life support will lessen the chance of a successful outcome.

The three elements of basic life support after initial assessment are commonly remembered as 'ABC'

AIRWAY   BREATHING   CIRCULATION

Assessment

○ Check whether the patient is responsive.

○ Shake gently by the shoulders and say loudly 'Are You All Right?'

If the patient responds by answering or moving the patient

○ Leave them in the position in which you find them (provided they are not in further danger) and check for any injury.

○ Reassess at intervals and go for help if help if needed.

If he is unresponsive:

○ Shout for help.

○ Open airway by tilting head and lifting chin.

○ Loosen any tight clothing around the neck.

○ Remove any obvious obstruction from the mouth, including loose dentures, but leave in place well-fitting dentures.

○ If possible with the patient in the position in which you find them, place your hand along the patient's hairline, exerting pressure to tilt the head.

○ With two fingers under the point of the chin, lift the chin – this will open the airway.

Look, listen and feel for breathing

○ Look for chest movements.

○ Listen at the mouth for breath sounds.

○ Feel for air with your cheek.

○ Look, listen and feel for up to ten seconds before deciding that breathing is absent.

If breathing is present place in the recovery position.

No breathing

○ Send for help or if you are on your own leave the patient and go and phone for the emergency services.

○ Return to the patient, check there is no obstruction; if there is an obstruction in the mouth turn the head to one side and scoop the obstruction out.

○ Ensure head tilt; chin lift.

○ Pinch the soft part of the patient's nose closed with index finger and thumb.

○ Allow the patient's mouth to open a little, but maintain chin lift.

○ Take a full breath and place your lips around the patient's mouth, making sure you have a good seal.

○ Breathe steadily into the mouth, watching for the chest to rise; it takes about two seconds for full inflation (if the chest does not rise it means either the seal around the mouth is not good, or the airway is obstructed. Check mouth seal and chin lift).

○ Taking your mouth away from the patient's, but continuing the head tilt; chin lift, allow the chest to fall passively as the air comes out. Take another full breath and repeat. Give two effective breaths.

Assess for signs of circulation

○ Look for any movement including swallowing or breathing.

○ Check the carotid pulse – take no more than ten seconds.

○ If you are confident that you can detect signs of circulation within ten seconds, continue rescue breathing until the victim starts breathing spontaneously, checking every 60 seconds that the pulse is still present.

○ When the patient starts to breathe for themselves, place into the recovery position and continue to monitor both pulse and breathing.

If there are no signs of a circulation, or you are at all unsure:

Start chest compression

○ Using your index and middle fingers, identify the lower rib margins. Keeping your fingers together, slide them upwards to the xiphisternum (the pointed end of the breast bone where the ribs meet).

○ With your middle finger over the xiphisternum, place your index finger on the bony sternum above.

○ Slide the heel of your hand down the sternum until it reaches your index finger; this should be the middle of the lower half of the sternum. Place the heel of your first hand on top of the other and interlock the fingers of both hands to ensure that pressure is not applied over the ribs.

○ Lean well over the patient, arms straight, and press down vertically on the sternum to depress it approximately 4 to 5 cms or one third of the chest cavity.

○ Release the pressure, then repeat at a rate of approximately 100 compressions a minute.

Now combine ventilation and compressions

○ After 15 compressions tilt the head, lift the chin and give two inflations.

○ Return your hands immediately to the sternum and give 15 further compressions.

○ Continue compressions and ventilation in a ratio of 15–2.

When to go for assistance

It is vital to get help as soon as possible. When more than one rescuer is available, one should start resuscitation while another gets help. A lone rescuer will have to decide whether to start resuscitation or go for help first.

In the following circumstances, or if the likely cause of unconsciousness is **drowning, trauma or the victim is an infant or child**, the rescuer should perform resuscitation for one minute before going for help.

If the victim is an adult and the cause of unconsciousness is not trauma or drowning, the rescuer should assume that the victim has a heart problem and go for help the instant it has been established that the victim is not breathing.

Pupils

Size of pupils is an unreliable sign of cardiac arrest and should not be used to influence management decisions.

Recovery position

When a patient is recovering and circulation and breathing have been restored, it is important to place the person in a position where the airway is protected and the risk of inhalation of gastric contents is minimised. The recovery position as described below enables this to take place, since it allows the head to be on a downward tilt, keeping the airway clear.

- Remove the patient's spectacles and bulky objects from their pockets.
- Kneel beside the patient and make sure that both their legs are straight.
- Open airway by tilting the head and lifting the chin.
- Place the arm nearest you out at right angles to the patient's body, elbow bent with the hand uppermost.
- Bring the far arm across the chest and hold the back of the hand against the cheek.
- With your other hand, grasp the far leg just above the knee and pull it up, keeping the foot on the ground.
- Keeping the hand pressed against the cheek, pull on the leg to roll the patient towards you onto their side.
- Adjust the upper leg so that both the hip and the knee are bent at right angles.
- Tilt the head back to ensure the airway remains open.
- Adjust the hand under the head to keep the head tilted if necessary.
- Check breathing and pulse regularly.

Method of turning patient onto their back

- Kneel by their side and place the arm nearest you above their head.
- Turn their head to face away from you.
- Grasp the patient's far shoulder with one hand and hip with the other, at the same time clamping the patient's wrist to the hip.
- With a steady pull roll the patient over against your thighs.
- Lower the patient gently to the ground on their back, supporting their head and shoulders as you do so; place the patient's extended arm by their side.

It is important to turn the patient over as quickly as possible whilst exercising great care, particularly not to injure their head.

☞ New guidelines issued discuss the possible inhibition of circulation to the underlying arm in the recovery position described. No definite ruling has however been made. The recovery position should be one that maintains and protects the airway, causing minimum discomfort to the patient.

Emergency/resuscitation drugs

OXYGEN	Breathing difficulties – lack of oxygen
ADRENALINE EPINEPHRINE	Cardiac arrest – anaphylactic shock
SALBUTAMOL	Bronchial dilator – asthma spasm
CHLORPHENIRAMINE	Antihistamine – allergies
HYDROCORTISONE	Anti-inflammatory – anaphylaxis – Addison collapse
MIDAZOLAM	Anticonvulsant – epilepsy – sedative
DEXTROSE	Diabetes – hypoglycaemia
DEXTROSE – INFUSION	Diabetes
ASPIRIN	Unstable angina – myocardial Infarction

Cardiac conditions

This section looks at:

❍ types of heart condition

❍ their causes and signs and symptoms

❍ principles of their management and treatment

❍ cardiac arrest

Many diseases affect the heart: they are classified according to the part they affect or the changes they produce. Management is often beyond the scope of the immediate carer, but you must be able to recognise life-threatening cardiac conditions and initiate care and assistance.

Aspects of modern living (smoking, alcohol consumption, sedentary lifestyle) have placed cardiac conditions very high among the main causes of death and the number of deaths is steadily rising.

Types of heart condition

The types of heart condition you are likely to confront will include the following.

Angina pectoris

Angina pectoris is a common condition. It is caused by reduced blood (and therefore oxygen) supply to the myocardium because of the narrowing of the coronary arteries in arteriosclerosis. This is a chronic condition that can bring on an acute attack.

Clinical signs

Quite often the pain is described as a heaviness in the arms or chest. Angina is often started by excessive exercise (e.g. digging, walking uphill, running).

○ Pain behind the breastbone, running the length of the bone and spreading across the chest.

○ Pain referred to the throat, jaw and teeth, the armpit and often into the left arm.

○ Short and sharp breathing.

○ Variable pulse.

○ Pallor.

People liable to angina attacks often carry GLYCERYL TRINITRATE for sub-lingual use.

Congestive heart failure

Congestive heart failure is a chronic condition occurring when the heart fails to pump adequately. It can have many causes:

1 myocardial infarction or ischaemic heart disease

2 hypertension

3 heart valve disease

Clinical signs

Because of the pulmonary congestion that results from left ventricular failure, the characteristic signs are respiratory. The usual signs are:

○ laboured breathing (dyspnoea)

○ sweating

○ cyanosis

○ ankle swelling

Severe respiratory discomfort is likely to occur when the patient is lying flat. These patients are often bedridden or unable to walk more than a few yards.

Management of cardiac conditions

○ Be calm and reassuring, do not leave the patient unattended.

○ Put the patient at rest, in a position that helps breathing.

○ Do not allow the patient to walk or make any unnecessary effort.

○ Reduce the work of the heart (exercise, emotions and excitement increase the heart action).

○ Keep the patient quiet and calm.

○ Loosen tight clothing.

○ Move patient as little as possible.

○ Give entonox (50% N_2O, 50% O_2) if pain is severe as with angina pectoris and myocardial infarction.

○ Arrange smooth removal to hospital.

○ Oxygen therapy will help with breathing – 6 litres per minute for an acute attack, 1–3 litres for a chronic attack.

☞ Be prepared to carry out CPR if needed.

These patients are usually very frightened. It is essential to reduce this fear. You can do this best by:

a a calm unhurried approach

b a confident manner, with plenty of reassurance

c providing a smooth comfortable transfer to hospital.

Myocardial infarction

A myocardial infarction (MI) occurs when a coronary artery or a branch of a coronary artery gets blocked. This is an 'acute' condition. The blockage (thrombosis) is often a blood clot or a fat embolism. This prevents the blood (and therefore the oxygen) from reaching the area of muscle beyond the blockage. This muscle eventually dies if the blood supply is not restored or if collateral circulation does not become established. The patient's survival depends on how much muscle is affected.

Clinical signs

The clinical signs will vary with the position and extent of the infarction and whether the electrical conduction system of the heart is affected. The usual signs are:

○ Severe central chest pains, which may radiate to one or both sides of the chest and into the neck, jaw or both arms.

○ Sudden onset of pain accompanied by sweating, faintness, giddiness, nausea, vomiting and fear of impending doom.

○ Shallow, painful breathing, greyness with cyanosis of the extremities.

○ Pupils may be slightly dilated.

○ Irregular pulse.

At first, patients often ignore these signs, especially if they are only slight, as they can be mistaken for indigestion.

Cardiac arrest DN01:3

Cardiac arrest is the sudden failure of the heart to pump sufficient blood to keep the brain alive. If the brain's blood supply is interrupted for more than three minutes it will certainly be irreversibly damaged. The brain only requires 1/6th of its normal supply of oxygen to protect it from damage.

The causes of cardiac arrest include: myocardial infarction; hypoxia (lack of oxygen); anaesthetic overdose; anaphylaxis; hypothermia; electrocution.

The signs of cardiac arrest include: loss of consciousness; absence of arterial pulse; absence of breathing; paleness/cyanosis; dilation and fixation of pupils.

ABSENCE OF A MAJOR PULSE IS THE DEFINITIVE DIAGNOSIS OF CARDIAC ARREST

Choking

This will be recognised by difficulty in breathing and speaking, possible cyanosis, gesturing and possible panic. The following measures should be taken:

○ Reassure.

○ Bend the patient forwards so that the head is lower than the chest.

○ Give five sharp blows between the shoulder blades with the flat of your hand.

○ If this fails try ABDOMINAL THRUSTS: sudden upward movement of the diaphragm compresses the chest and may clear the obstruction.

○ If this fails try again FOUR MORE TIMES, ALTERNATING BETWEEN FIVE BACK BLOWS WITH FIVE THRUSTS.

○ If the patient loses consciousness muscle spasm may be relieved. Check to see if breathing has started. If not, turn on to side and give four to five blows between the shoulder blades.

○ If this fails kneel astride the patient and give abdominal thrusts.

○ If breathing starts, place in the recovery position, call an ambulance and check breathing and pulse continuously.

○ If breathing ceases DIAL 999 and perform life support procedures.

In an unconscious patient, ventilate between back thrusts and abdominal trusts. It is possible that sufficient oxygen may be administered, preventing the heart from becoming hypoxic and arresting. More importantly you will know if the obstruction has been removed from the airway, but may not have been expelled.

Infant under one year

○ Lay the baby along your forearm.

○ Check mouth.

○ Five back blows.

○ Five chest thrusts.

○ NO ABDOMINAL THRUSTS.

Infant over one, under five years

○ Place the child over the knee, head down.

○ Check mouth.

○ Five back blows.

○ Five chest thrust or five abdominal thrusts.

Any patient who has received abdominal thrusts or had severe obstruction removed should be examined at hospital for either possible internal injury through the abdominal thrusts or by particles of the obstruction having entered the lungs, where, if left, it will cause inflammation.

Faint

Fainting is the most common cause of sudden loss of consciousness. About two per cent of patients faint before, during or after dental treatment. Young fit adult males are especially prone to faint in the dental surgery – especially after injections. The causes of fainting include: anxiety; pain; fatigue; fasting; high temperature and relative humidity.

The patient's symptoms include: dizziness; weakness; and nausea.

The clinical signs include:

○ Pulse – slow and feeble, changing to feeble and fast.

○ Skin – cold and clammy.

○ Colour – pale.

○ Pupils – equal and dilated.

○ Breathing – feeble and shallow.

The treatment procedure is:

○ Lay the patient down.

○ Elevate the legs.

○ Loosen any tight clothing.

○ Ensure good air supply and clear airway.

○ If unconscious, place in recovery position.

○ Monitor patient until they recover fully.

○ Be alert to any changes of condition.

☞ If recovery is not rapid then other causes of collapse must be considered, i.e. anaphylaxis, hypoglycaemia, myocardial infarction.

Asthma

Asthma is a narrowing of the bronchioles due to a spasm of the bronchi muscles. There is usually an allergic cause, but respiratory infection or stress will often bring on an acute attack. The signs and symptoms of asthma include:

○ Wheezing due to difficulty in exhaling through narrow constricted airways.

○ Laboured breathing as the patient finds the actual process of breathing demands great effort.

○ Oxygen deficiency as the attack progresses.

Management

○ **NEVER LAY THE PATIENT FLAT**

○ Allow patient to assume a position that is most comfortable for them.

○ Allow access to inhaler.

○ Reassure patient – give oxygen at the rate of 6/8 litres per minute if required.

○ If attack does not respond quickly – summon help.

Epilepsy (Range e)

Epilepsy is a common illness usually characterised by convulsions (a fit) during which the patient is unconscious. The fit is caused by abnormal electrical activity in the brain. Although frightening to witness, epileptic convulsions are not usually life threatening to the patient.

Types of epilepsy

Petit mal
Characterised by brief lapses of awareness.

Grand mal
Classic convulsion – more severe.

Status epileptic
Continuous convulsion.

Signs and symptoms
❍ Loss of consciousness.

❍ Rigid extended body, cyanosis may occur and lasts about 30 seconds.

❍ Uncontrolled jerking movements.

❍ Sometimes incontinent.

❍ Convulsion gradually stops, patient may sleep.

Management
❍ Protect patient from injuring him/herself.

❍ Protect and maintain airway.

❍ Give oxygen.

❍ **DO NOT PUT ANYTHING IN PATIENT'S MOUTH**.

❍ Patients may sleep after a convulsion – this is normal, treat as for unconscious.

❍ Summon help.

❍ Give reassurance and emotional support to patient and relatives.

In status epilepsy, diazepam or midazolam may be given by IV or IM by trained medical or clinical staff to control multiple convulsion.

Diabetes
Diabetes is a disorder in which the pancreas fails to produce enough insulin for carbohydrate metabolism. Glucose absorbed from the gastro-intestinal tract cannot be adequately metabolised or stored and so reaches higher than normal levels in the bloodstream.

Hypoglycaemia
This is a diabetic emergency caused by the patient having too much insulin activity. The patient may have missed a meal or overdosed on insulin therapy. The most common cause is increased muscular exercise reducing the blood sugar to abnormal levels. The onset of hypoglycaemia is often very sudden. The signs include:

❍ Onset – minutes

❍ Skin – profuse sweating and pale colour

○ Breathing – normal to shallow

○ Pulse – fast and full 100+

○ Breath odour – none

○ Physical signs – may be uncoordinated, confused, aggressive.

Hyperglycaemia

This is excessively high levels of glucose in the blood, the result of poor diabetic control and is most common in insulin-dependent diabetics. Treatment requires rehydration with infusion fluids – therefore hospitalisation is required. The signs include:

○ Onset – gradual, hours to days

○ Skin – dry and flushed

○ Breathing – deep and sighing

○ Pulse – fast 100+

○ Breath odour – sweet and fruity (acetone)

○ Physical signs – restlessness, drowsiness, lethargic.

Management

There is often confusion between hyPOglycaemia and hypERglycaemia. If in doubt give oral glucose – it will do no harm to the hypER but will rapidly reverse the hyPO.

☞ **HypO is the Greek word for too LITTLE**

HypER is the Greek word for too MUCH

Anaphylactic shock DN01:3

Anaphylactic shock is the body's exaggerated response to a foreign antigenic substance.

Anaphylaxis is mediated by antibodies, which cause histamines and other vaso-active mediators to be released from cells of the body causing circulatory, cutaneous and gastro-intestinal effects. Anaphylactoid **reactions** present in a similar manner to shock but there is no previous sensitisation. The treatment is the same.

SUDDEN COLLAPSE AND DEATH CAN RESULT

Certain patients are more susceptible to anaphylaxis, such as asthmatics and chronic hayfever sufferers. There is, however, no way of being sure that an anaphylactic shock is not going to occur. The fact that they are comparatively rare means that it is all the more important that the clinical signs can be quickly recognised, as the condition responds well to prompt diagnosis.

Signs and symptoms

○ Flushing of skin

○ Laryngeal oedema (swelling of the vocal cords resulting in airway obstruction)

○ Bronchospasm

○ Hypotension (drop in blood pressure)

○ Cardiovascular collapse associated with vasodilation and an increase in vascular permeability.

Management

○ 1–1000 adrenaline Epinephrine 0.5ml – 1ml intramuscular

○ Administer oxygen

○ Chlorpheniramine 10 – 20mg IM repeated if required or Slow IV 10–20mg diluted in syringe with 5–10ml sterile water for injection

○ 200mg hydrocortisone IV

○ Intravenous fluids

○ Arrange transfer to hospital immediately

○ Prepare for emergency intubation or cricoidthyrotomy.

☞ **ALWAYS BE PREPARED FOR A CARDIAC ARREST**

Drug administration table for anaphylaxis

INTERMUSCULAR ADRENALINE
 	
1 in 1000
	ADULT CHILD
	
	0.5 – 1ml 1yr 0.1 ml
	
	                3/4yr 0.3ml
	
	                5yr 0.4ml
	
	                10yr 0.5ml
	
	Repeat after 10 minutes if no improvement

INTRAVENOUS ADRENALINE EPINEPHRINE 1 in 10.000	**Used with extreme caution** 5ml / 1.10,000 at a rate = 100mcg/ 1ml per minute
OXYGEN	4 to 6 litres per minute
INTRAVASCULAR VOLUME EXPANSION (if available)	Preferably colloid in a dose of; 10ml/kg given rapidly
SALBUTAMOL BY NEBULIZER	
ANTIHISTAMINE AND STEROIDS	No immediate effect but may be beneficial later
CHLORPHENIRAMINE (piriton) 10–20 mgs IM 1yr 2 mg 7yr 5 mg 12yr 10 mg	Slow IV Chlorpheniramine may be given 10–20mgs diluted in syringe with 5–10ml sterile water for injection
HYDROCORTISONE	200mg 50–100mg intravenously

Shock

☞ **DEAL WITH SHOCK QUICKLY BEFORE IT KILLS**

Shock can be divided into three categories.

○ Cardiogenic

○ Hypovolaemic

○ Anaphylactic

Each form of shock can prove fatal and therefore needs to be managed as quickly as possible.

Cardiogenic
Interruption of the heart's normal electrical pacemaker, e.g. bad news, electrocution, visual shock, pain.

Hypovolaemic
Loss of body fluids through dehydration, blood loss, excessive peripheral perfusion.

Anaphylactic
An excessive reaction of the body to a foreign substance, e.g. bee sting, drugs, food.

Early Development	Loss of Compensation	Late Development
Increased pulse rate	Skin colour changes	Changes in levels of consciousness
Increased respiration	Rapid weak pulse	Marked drop in blood pressure
Restlessness	Laboured breathing	Weak pulse
Fearfulness	Weakness	Weakened respiration
Increased capillary	Thirstiness	Unconsciousness
Refill time	Nausea	

Emergency guidelines
REMEMBER: **A** – ASSESS PATIENT AND CHECK AIRWAY

B – BREATHING

C – CIRCULATION

Cause of Collapse	Signs/Symptoms	Treatment
Fainting	Pallor, Sweating, Cold, Nausea	Head down tilt Oxygen
Anaphylaxis	Bronchospasm, Drop in BP, Rash	Adrenaline O_2 Hydrocortisone Chlopheniramine
Hypoglycaemia	Confusion, Pallor, Aggression, Coma	Oral/IV Glucose Glucagon
Epilepsy	Aura, Muscular spasms	Protect patient Oxygen
Respiratory obstruction	Cyanosis, See-saw breathing	Clear blockage Oxygen
Asthma	Wheezing bronchospasm	Salbutamol inhaler/nebuliser/oxygen
Myocardial infarction	Severe pain in chest, Pallor	N_2O/O_2 or O_2 Allow patient to sit semi-reclined
Heart attack	Difficulty in breathing	Consider 300mg Aspirin if not contra indicated
Angina	Chest pain	Glyceryl Trinitrate sublingual Oxygon
CVA stroke	Confusion, Muscle weakness Speech problems Unconscious	O_2 Reassure patient

 IF THE PATIENT DOES NOT RESPOND SEEK ASSISTANCE 999

CROSS INFECTION CONTROL 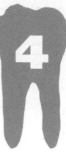 4

Introduction

This chapter is linked to DN02 of the NVQ Level 3 in Oral Health Care and looks at ways in which cross infection can be prevented in the dental surgery by the dental team.

Cross infection is the transmission of micro-organisms, spores and viruses, this can be by:

○ Droplet infection, e.g. coughing, sneezing, speech

○ Unsterilised instruments

○ Contaminated gloves or hands.

An example of this is shown in the diagram below

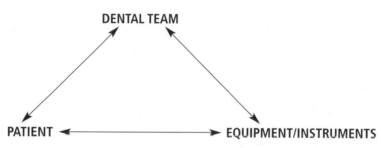

The dentist has the major responsibility for liability. This responsibility is to ensure that all proper precautions are implemented to protect and safeguard the dental team and the patients who attend for dental treatment. Precautions must be set in place to protect individuals from health hazards.

The workplace must have a Health and Safety Policy that includes:

○ An infection control policy

○ An at risk assessment policy

○ Control of substances hazardous to health (COSHH) document.

The General Dental Council (GDC) covers dental practices, dentists and the dental team within the workplace. The dentist and dental team are legally obliged to co-operate fully with the Infection Control Policy. Protocols must be followed in relation to Health and Safety and Risk Assessment, which should include:

○ Vaccination of all the dental team against Hepatitis B

○ The wearing of Protective Personal Equipment (PPE)

○ Zoning (a designed clean and dirty area)

○ The use of sterilisation for all instruments

○ Disposal of sharps, e.g. needles, scalpel blades by the operator

○ Correct disposal of waste.

QUESTIONS

? Question 1

a. Where do you keep your Health and Safety Policy?

_____

_____

b. When was the last entry made?

_____

_____

The workplace

The layout of the surgery should be simple and uncluttered. The surgery should be well ventilated and, if necessary, ventilation systems should be provided if windows do not provide sufficient ventilation.

The surgery walls should be easy to clean with no cracks or joins. The floor covering should be one complete unit with sealed joins between the floor and the walls. This should not be a carpet. The door handles and light switches should be easy to use and clean. The surgery should have drawer and cupboard handles that can be easily disinfected. The surface of the dental chair should be smooth with no joins or cracks. Preferably the switches should be operated by the foot.

Preparation of the workplace

The dental nurse (DN) should ensure that the surfaces in the surgery are cleaned on a daily basis. This is called surgery hygiene. The surgery should be cleaned in between patients and after treatment has been completed. The surfaces should be washed with the use of an enzyme-based detergent solution and napkin, or a similar cleansing solution. This will include:

○ the bracket table, handpiece connection leads

○ worktops and cupboard surfaces that may collect dust

○ the stools used by the dentist and the DN

○ the dental chair, the dental light and handles on the dental light

○ aspirator connections together with the tubing

○ the spittoon should be the last item to be wiped with the napkin, which then should be disposed of in a yellow clinical waste bag.

When all the areas have been washed the DN should put disposable plastic coverings on all the areas that the dentist and DN will touch. The plastic coverings can be sticky or made in such a way that they will stay in place once put into position. The areas concerned are:

○ handles that may be touched by the dentist, for example

   – the bracket table

   – the dental overhead light

○ the section of the dental chair where the patient rests their head

○ the light curing machine

○ during a surgical procedure all the lines from the bracket table should be covered, as this will prevent contamination from blood and saliva.

It is important that the plastic coverings are removed and disposed of after each patient has completed treatment and left the surgery. The plastic coverings are disposed of in the yellow clinical waste bags.

Air and water lines

The air and water lines connected to the bracket table should be flushed through for a period of at least three minutes in the morning and for at least 30 seconds in between patients. This is done to ensure that any back flow of water has been removed from the lines before commencing treatment on the next patient.

Dental records

To avoid contamination, dental records and radiographs should be handled without gloves on, but hands must be clean.

Zoning

Another aid to prevent cross infection in the workplace is the use of clearly marked 'clean' and 'dirty' areas. This is commonly known as zoning. The 'clean' area should be used for freshly sterilised items; the 'dirty' area should be used for used instruments awaiting sterilisation.

During treatment it is imperative that no member of the dental team touches the 'clean' area with contaminated gloves or the 'dirty' area with clean gloves. It is the DN's responsibility to ensure that the dentist does not enter 'clean' areas with contaminated gloves. Don't forget gloves are contaminated before treatment commences, during the oral examination. Both the dentist and the DN should continually remember to remove contaminated gloves when entering clean areas. It is paramount in the continual quest for reducing cross infection.

Waste disposal

Dentists have a legal obligation to dispose of clinical waste, without risk to the dental team, patients and the public. Clinical waste should never be disposed of through the domestic waste system.

Aspirators and tubing should be cleaned regularly in accordance with the manufacturer's instructions. Aspirator tips should be disposed of or sterilised after use.

Infected waste, e.g. blood, saliva, suction waste, should be put into a system that is connected to a sanitary sewer system. Heavy-duty gloves, protective eye wear, a mask and protective clothing should be worn by the dental team when disposing of such waste.

Clinical bags

○ Yellow plastic bags are used for clinical waste, e.g. swabs, cotton wool rolls. Ideally the bag should be placed in a foot-operated bin.

○ Black plastic bags are used for paper waste only.

○ Clothes bags are used for dental coats and sent to a laundry, or an industrial company may be used.

Disposal of amalgam

Waste amalgam must be placed in specially designed containers in the workplace and collected by an approved disposal firm on a regular basis.

Question 2

a. How do you prepare your workplace in the morning?

_____

b. How are clinical waste products disposed of within your workplace?

_____

c. What happens to the dirty laundry in your workplace?

_____

Disposal of sharps

○ All sharps must be disposed of in a rigid sharps container, which must be clearly labelled.

○ Local anaesthetic solution should be placed in a separate sharps bin.

○ If possible take the sharps bin to the operator for the removal of sharps.

○ The sharps bin should be between 4ft (1.22m) and 4ft 6 (1.37m) off the floor, preferably on a purpose-built bracket on the wall.

○ When the sharps bin is two-thirds full, the bin should be securely sealed and arrangements made for collection and incineration.

○ Disposal of waste must be undertaken by an appropriate waste disposal firm. It is the dentist's legal responsibility to ensure that the firm is registered with a Waste Control Authority, which complies with existing regulations.

Sharps injury

A written policy describing the management of sharps injuries should be displayed in a prominent position in the workplace. Recommended procedures following a sharps injury are as follows:

○ Rinse the area under cold running water

○ Encourage bleeding

○ Cover the area with a waterproof dressing

○ Inform the dentist/supervising DN

○ Record the incident.

A first aid station should be in each workplace and should contain:

○ a first aid box

○ an eye station containing sterile eye wash

○ an ambu bag.

The employee has a duty to:

RIDDOR STANDS FOR THE REPORTING OF INJURIES, DISEASES AND DANGEROUS OCCURRENCES – RIDDOR REGULATIONS 1995

○ Report any injury/accident at work

○ Obtain treatment if necessary

○ Keep the employer informed of any after-effects, including sick leave.

The employer has a duty to:

○ Investigate the circumstances of the incident and address if required

○ Keep a record of all reported incidents

○ Liaise with medical personnel.

COSHH STANDS FOR THE CONTROL OF SUBSTANCES HAZARDOUS TO HEALTH

The COSHH 1999 Regulations state that the employer is responsible:

'for preventing or adequately controlling exposure of its employees to hazardous substances through a systematic process of identifying hazards, assessing significant risks and introducing control measures.'

Impressions

Impressions should be rinsed and disinfected before sending to the laboratory. Impressions should be immersed in a disinfectant for ten minutes, always follow the manufacturer's instructions. Impressions should then be put in self-seal plastic bags before sending to the laboratory. Alginate impressions should be kept moist with damp gauze. The laboratory card must be clearly filled in stating the patient's name, date, work required and the date due back.

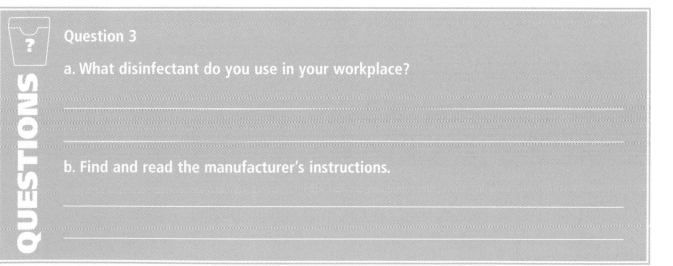

QUESTIONS

Question 3

a. What disinfectant do you use in your workplace?

b. Find and read the manufacturer's instructions.

Personal Protection Equipment

A high level of personal hygiene is vital for cross infection control. When working with patients the DN should refrain from touching anything that is not required for the treatment. Hair should be worn off the face.

Uniform

It is the responsibility of all the dental team to ensure that their uniforms are clean, neat and appropriately worn. A short sleeve top and trousers are recommended. Uniforms should be changed daily or more often if they have become contaminated with blood or other materials. Shoes should be flat and covered in to protect the feet.

Glasses

Protective glasses or visors should be worn to protect the DN from infection and debris.

Gloves

Gloves must always be worn when treating patients:

○ A new pair of gloves should be used for each patient

○ Gloves must never be washed or reused

○ Gloves must be changed if punctured.

Masks

Masks should be worn during dental treatment and should be changed for each patient.

Hand washing

It is important for all the dental team to ensure that they have washed their hands in the correct manner stipulated by the Health and Safety Council. This should be carried out by all the dental staff before treatment commences, using the correct skin cleanser. A suitable pump dispenser should be provided. It is the dentist's legal responsibility to provide all materials and equipment within the workplace for the dental team and the patient's protection.

○ Care of hands is vital to infection control. Skin that is lacerated, abraded or cracked can offer a very good point of entry for micro-organisms.

○ Any open skin wounds or cuts should be covered with a suitable waterproof dressing, this should be shown to the dentist/supervising DN who will give the all clear to proceed or not.

○ Care of the skin is helped with the regular use of a good emollient hand cream to prevent skin from drying out. Hand cream should be used after washing the hands when the clinical session has ended.

○ Before hand washing, all jewellery – rings with gemstones, bracelets and watches should be removed. Wedding rings without gemstones can be worn, but should be removed if possible to ensure that the hands are totally free from any major foreign bodies resident either under the ring or on the skin of the hand.

○ Hand washing should be performed in a careful and methodical manner using a suitable skin disinfectant. A full hand wash is recommended before glove protection can be worn.

○ The taps in the surgery should have handles that ideally can be operated by the elbows. These taps are operated without having to personally touch them with the hands in order to turn them on or off. If elbow-operated taps are not available the DN should ensure that the taps are washed daily and are kept as clean as possible in between patients.

○ Once the water has been mixed to a warm temperature the use of a suitable cleanser should be introduced.

The DN should take particular care under the nails of the hands, which should be kept as short as possible. The nails should be free of nail varnish and nail extensions. This is to ensure that any underlining debris found under the fingernail is kept to the bare minimum.

○ Hand washing should be carried out for at least 30 seconds.

○ The fingers, hands, wrists and the lower arm below the elbow should be washed.

○ When the hand washing has been completed the arms should be rinsed, letting the water run from the fingers to the hand and elbow.

○ The DN should ensure that the water does not flow back down the arm to the hand or the fingers. The arm should be kept as upright as possible. If water is allowed to flow back down the arm to the hand, it will result in recontamination of the skin and the whole procedure will have to be redone.

○ After the hands have been washed they should be dried with a clean disposable paper towel.

Aseptic technique
See Chapter 11

QUESTIONS

?

Question 3

What type of solution do you use to wash your hands in your workplace?

_____

_____

_____

_____

Patient protection
Protective glasses and a disposable bib should be used to protect the patient against debris, splashes and materials.

Methods of sterilisation
Prior to sterilisation, instruments should be scrubbed under cold running water to remove all debris. This is achieved by using a long-handled brush with liquid soap whilst wearing heavy-duty gloves. An ultrasonic bath would perform a similar function. On removal from the bath the instruments are dried and placed loosely on a perforated tray in the autoclave.

The autoclave
The autoclave is the most common form of sterilisation in the workplace and is worked by steam under pressure similar to a pressure cooker. Following cleaning, instruments should be loosely placed on a perforated tray. Each morning the chamber has to be filled to the

required limit with distilled water and emptied at the end of each day. Hand pieces can be autoclaved, but must be lubricated beforehand. It is advised to refer to a manufacturer's guide or the Medical Devices Agency (MDA).

The autoclave must be serviced regularly to ensure it is functioning correctly.

Colour change indicators used when autoclaving merely tell us that it is temperature sensitive, it is not an indication that the load is sterile. The monitoring of autoclaves is essential. Most have a printout to record each stage of the process. Autoclaves must be timed by the DN each day to make sure the minimum time of three minutes has occurred.

Advantages
- Kills all known micro organisms, spores and viruses
- Suitable for most dental instruments
- Sterilisation time 3 minutes at 134°C
- Complete cycle approximately 15 minutes
- Cannot open the door during the cycle.

Disadvantages
- Not suitable for plastic instruments.

Glass bead steriliser
These are used at the chairside for momentarily sterilising reamers and files during root canal treatment. The glass beads are heated up to a temperature of 265°C. The endodontic instruments are placed in the glass beads for 10 seconds and then inserted into the root canal.

Industrial sterilisation
Certain items used in the dental surgery are sterilised using gamma irradiation, e.g. sutures, dental needles, scalpel blades. These are all packaged sterile and are for single use only. Gamma irradiation kills off all viruses, spores, fungi and bacteria. This process cannot be undertaken in the dental surgery, as it requires the use of elaborate equipment. A microbiological test is carried out with each load, which takes about 7–10 days to confirm that sterilisation has taken place. The spore test should read negative. Once items have been put through this process using ethylene oxide gas they must be held in bond for varying periods to allow the gas to vent.

Central sterile supply department
The instruments are sterilised in a high vacuum porous load autoclave. Hospitals use this method of sterilisation. The dirty instruments are collected by the CSSD staff and returned sterile packaged and placed in a clean area. This system can only work by duplicating the number of instruments used.

Latex allergy
In recent years it has been reported that latex allergy is on the increase. In the most extreme cases a person will have an anaphylactic shock that could prove fatal.

Other symptoms might include urticaria, redness, swelling, sneezing, wheezing and coughing. Most dental products contain latex, although latex-free products are now available. These include:

- Examination gloves
- Rubber dam
- Mouth props
- Local anaesthetic cartridges
- Disposable syringes.

Preparing the surgery

Care must be taken when preparing the surgery for patients allergic to latex. Known latex allergy patients should be treated at the beginning of a treatment session, as throughout the day there may be high levels of aerosolised latex products in the ambient air. All latex products must be removed and placed in another room or stored in a cupboard.

The surgery must be washed using latex-free gloves, with a liquid detergent to clear away all dirt and dust. The patient's case notes must be clearly labelled Latex Allergy. Dental treatment can be carried out successfully if such precautions are adhered to.

If it is not known that the patient has an allergy to latex and suddenly becomes ill within minutes of exposure, management of the patient should be as follows:

- In the case of a medical emergency, the surgery must be equipped with the relevant first aid items and drugs including Adrenaline.
- An ambulance must be called for whilst the dentist deals with the immediate emergency.
- All products contained in the first aid box must be latex-free.

Depending on the severity of the reaction, four stages have been identified:

1 Localised contact urticaria (itching)

2 Generalised urticaria, including swelling.

3 Urticaria and symptoms of mucous membranes.

4 Anaphylactic shock reaction.

QUESTIONS

Question 4

Why is it important to treat a patient that is allergic to latex at the beginning of a treatment session?

Hepatitis B

Hepatitis B is an inflammation of the liver caused by a virus. This virus is usually spread by contact with infected blood, such as blood transfusions or hypodermic needles that are shared with drug users, and sexual contact.

The Hepatitis B virus has been found in all body fluids including blood, saliva and breast milk. Symptoms of Hepatitis B are:

○ Jaundice (but not in every case)

○ Weakness

○ Loss of appetite

○ Nausea

○ Brownish urine, pale bowel movements

○ Abdominal discomfort.

It is possible for a person to be infected with the virus but not to have any symptoms of the disease. Such people are known as carriers and they may also be unaware that they are carriers. Vaccination is the best protection against Hepatitis B. This requires three injections of the vaccine. All healthcare workers must be vaccinated against HBV and this is usually done before they start work and come into contact with patients.

Universal precautions apply to all patients, whether they have a blood-borne virus or not, in the dental surgery.

Hepatitis C

Hepatitis C is a virus that can damage the liver. There is no vaccination for Hepatitis C and, like Hepatitis B, it is carried in the blood. It has also been detected in other body fluids. Hepatitis C is spread by the sharing of needles for injecting drugs and receiving a blood transfusion (before September 1991). Needles and syringes are the greatest risk of infection.

Symptoms of Hepatitis C are:

○ Nausea, loss of appetite

○ Muscle aches and high temperature

○ Weight loss

○ Mild jaundice

○ Joint pain

○ Fatigue

○ Depression and anxiety.

A person that has the virus may not actually show any signs or symptoms for years, even decades, but the virus can still be passed to others. About 1 in 5 people that have the virus will develop severe liver damage. This is known as cirrhosis. As there is no vaccine for Hepatitis C it is highly probable that patients will be treated in the dental surgery without knowing they are carriers. Therefore, universal precautions apply to all patients whether they have any blood-borne virus or not.

HIV & AIDS

AIDS, or Acquired Immune Deficiency Syndrome, is a disease that destroys some of the body's white blood cells, leaving the body's natural defence system impaired.

HIV is Human Immunodeficiency Virus, which is a virus that attacks the T4 lymphocyte white cell in the blood. Firstly it multiplies inside the cell when penetrated, takes over the nuclear material and uses it to make more virus particles. The cell then dies, releasing new virus particles into the blood to infect more cells.

HIV is spread by having unprotected sex and sharing needles for drug use. Symptoms can be

○ Short feverish illness

○ Swollen glands and occasionally the virus may cause symptoms of meningitis.

A person with those symptoms may not realise that they are infected with HIV. Often the first sign of chronic infection is a condition called PGL. This is Persistent Generalised Lymphadenopathy. This condition affects the back of the neck and under the arms. Other symptoms that may develop are:

○ Fever

○ Loss of weight

○ Candida (thrush)

○ Infections of the mouth

○ Attacks of diarrhoea.

Dental treatment for patients with HIV should be the same as for all other patients, using universal precautions.

QUESTIONS

Question 5

a. What is meant by universal precautions?

_____

_____

b. Name two other blood-borne viruses.

_____

_____

Creutzfeldt-Jakob disease

Creutzfeldt-Jakob disease (CJD) is a rapidly progressive neurodegenerative disorder, which is invariably fatal. The average age of onset is between 55 and 75 years old.

A related condition known as variant CJD, which is similar to CJD, has a peak incidence much lower, around the age of 27. The vast majority of patients with CJD usually die within one year of illness onset. The Spongiform Encephalopathy Advisory Committee (SEAC) monitors CJD.

Scientists say that there is a theoretical risk that CJD could be passed on by contaminated surgical instruments in dentistry. SEAC has warned that CJD cannot be completely inactivated by sterilisation. There is concern about the fact that Creutzfeldt-Jakob disease may not be completely inactivated by sterilisation. Dentists must use universal infection control procedures for all patients and be aware of future developments regarding this disease.

It is important to note that there has not been a single case in the UK of the disease being transmitted by surgical instruments (verified by British Dental Association on 1/11/02).

MRSA

MRSA stands for Methicillin Resistant *Staphylococcus Aureus*. *Staphylococcus Aureus* is a bacterium that can be found in about 20–30 per cent of healthy people. This bacterium lives in the nose, throat and on the skin. Staphylococcus Aureus that is resistant to antibiotics including Methicillin becomes known as MRSA.

People that have MRSA are commonly patients that are already in hospital and are usually found in wards such as surgical, orthopaedic, burns units and intensive care. Hospital staff and members of the public need not be overly concerned with MRSA as it is confined mainly to those patients that are debilitated.

KEY WORDS

Colonisation of MRSA. This means the presence of the organism on the skin, nose or throat of people without illness.

Infected with MRSA. This is when there is fever and inflammation occurring in the presence of MRSA.

Colonisation of Staff is treated by using topical agents and also special antibiotics. Bathing and hair washing is done with chlorhexadine. Infection is treated with certain types of antibiotics by intravenous infusion, which may be toxic. Therefore, patients that are infected must be treated in hospital.

Hand washing prevents the spread of MRSA. Staff in hospitals must be scrupulous when hand washing before and after contact with patients. This is the most important infection control factor and also patient notes must be clearly labelled MRSA so that the patients can be isolated in a room. If this is not possible, then the patient should be nursed in a ward away from other non-infected patients. Regular damp dusting is recommended if the patient is isolated and the door must be closed.

QUESTIONS

Question 6

Is it possible for someone to be colonised with MRSA without them actually knowing?

References for latex allegies
S. M. Hashim Nainar, *Journal of Paediatric Dentistry 2001*.

References for Hepatitis B
Smith, Dr T (ed): *The New Macmillan Guide to Family Health*; Macmillan, 1989.

References for HIV & AIDS
Macmillan Family Health (Dr Tony Smith).

References for CJD
British Dental Association, 64 Wimpole Street, London, W1G 8YS; www.bda-dentistry.org.uk

The Department of Health, Richmond House, 79 Whitehall, London, SW1A 2NL; www.doh.gov.uk

US Department of Health and Human Services, see www.health.state.ny.us

5 DENTAL RADIOGRAPHY

Dental Nurses who possess the accredited post-qualification certificate in Dental Radiography[1] are permitted to take certain dental radiographs in the dental surgery, but this chapter simply addresses the role and the diverse responsibilities of the dental nurse in supporting the production of dental radiographs in the dental surgery. The following topics will be covered:

- Ionising radiation
- X-ray production
- Radiation protection
- Clinical governance
- Legislation
- Principles of dental radiography
- Preparation of equipment (DN14.1)
- Preparation and management of patients (DN14.1)
- Cross infection (DN14.1)
- Film processing and darkroom practice (DN14.1)
- Film mounting (DN14.2)
- Quality assurance and film fault analysis (DN14.1 & DN14.3)
- Health and safety and risk assessment (DN14.3).

Ionising radiation

X-rays are found at the high energy/short-wavelength end of the electromagnetic spectrum, somewhere between ultra-violet and gamma rays.

Properties of X-rays:

- Travel in straight lines
- Penetrate matter
- Can induce changes in living tissue and genetic effects
- Will scatter once their energy is attenuated as a result of interaction with matter
- Not detected by human senses, e.g., not seen, felt or heard
- Produce a latent image on photographic or x-ray film.

For protection purposes it is useful to know that, like light, X-rays travel in straight lines. Thus X-rays emitted from a point source diverge and the intensity is inversely proportional to the square of the distance travelled. This relationship is known as the inverse square law.[2]

Certain harmful biological effects are associated with exposure to ionising radiation:

(a) Somatic effects – this term is derived from the Greek word *soma* meaning body and refers to the effects directly suffered by the body of the individual who has been exposed to ionising radiation. These can be either 'deterministic effects,'[3] those which are always associated with exposure to high levels of radiation ranging from erythema (reddening of the skin) through to cataracts in the lens of the eye, depending on the dose received above a certain threshold below which no effects will be seen, or 'stochastic effects,'[4] which develop randomly in response to radiation doses. The likelihood of the effects, which include solid tumours or leukaemia, becomes greater with increasing dose. The patient dose involved in dental radiography is usually very small but it is essential to keep operator, as well as patient dose, to a minimum in order to avoid development of any undesirable effects.[5]

(b) Genetic effects – it is generally considered that exposures to high levels of radiation can potentially result in damage to genes, leading to the possibility of abnormality in the next generation.

When considering an individual's exposure to ionising radiation, it is important to remember that we are not just talking about their exposure to medical radiation from X-rays, nuclear medicine or radiotherapy, but also to background radiation naturally occurring in the environment, i.e. cosmic radiation or radiation that is emitted from radioactive minerals such as uranium present in granite.[6]

X-ray production

X-rays are produced by means of a high current being passed across a wire filament causing electrons to be emitted (see Figure 5.1). This process is known as *thermionic emission*. A negative charge is applied to the focusing cup and because like charges repel each other this focuses the negatively charged electrons into a fine stream. A high potential difference (usually between 60 and 70 KV in modern units) accelerates the electrons across the tube to hit the tungsten anode. It is important that the X-ray tube is a vacuum otherwise the electrons would collide with air molecules. The energy of the electrons is converted into 2 per cent X-rays and 98 per cent heat. The angulation of the anode means that any X-rays travelling in the wrong direction will be absorbed by the anode and those travelling in the right direction leave through a small port in the outer metal casing and are further collimated by the metal cone.

Scatter radiation results when X-rays pass through matter so that their energy is partly attenuated, which results in them changing direction. Although low energy radiation makes no positive contribution to the image, it contributes to the patient dose. Some of the low energy radiation produced by the X-ray tube is attenuated by the oil and glass, but to further improve the quality of the beam, filtration equivalent of up to 2mm of aluminium is added. Beam limiting devices help to minimise the effect of scatter on the film.

A brief explanation of the process may help to reassure the patient, however, questions relating to diagnosis or requiring more detailed answers should be referred to the clinician. (DN14.1).

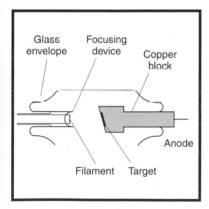

Figure 5.1: Diagram of an X-ray tube.

Radiation protection

The Ionising Radiation Regulations for Medical Exposures 2000 (IR(ME)R 2000) is a legal document that lays down basic measures for protection from medical radiation exposures, including who is entitled to justify the exposure and who is allowed to work as an operator. The regulations demand written employer's procedures (for example, who is allowed to refer patients for X-ray) and written protocols to ensure good and safe practice. These regulations are law and must not be breached. The Ionising Radiations Regulations 1999 (IRR99) lays down measures for the protection of staff and public from the dangers of ionising radiation. This would include the proper use and maintenance of X-ray and processing equipment. The IRR99 also requires the drawing up of local rules for radiation safety.

Protective measures include:

○ The operator must be properly trained and must undergo regular continuing professional development (CPD) to remain competent.

○ All exposures must be justified in order to balance the benefit to the patient with any risk involved and sufficient information needs to be recorded on the X-ray request form for this to be done.

○ A controlled area around the X-ray equipment should be designated and access to this area must be prohibited when radiography is being carried out.

○ Non-essential personnel should remain outside the controlled area while the exposure is made.[7]

○ The operator should stand a minimum of 2 m from the X-ray tube or within 'a protected area.'[8]

○ Open-ended rectangular collimation must be used for bitewings and periapicals.

○ Beam aiming devices must be used for bitewings and periapical films.[9]

○ Quality assurance programmes with written protocols must be in place to review image quality and reject analysis, processing and the performance of X-ray equipment to optimise exposures and keep dose to the patient as low as reasonably practicable.[10] (DN14.1and DN14.3)

○ The National Radiological Protection Board (NRPB) recommend that the tube output should be greater than 50 KV and ideally within the 60–70 KV range.[11]

○ Exposures should be kept as low as reasonably practicable and this can be achieved through the use of F-speed film or digital radiography.

○ Check if there is any likelihood that the patient could be pregnant.[12]

○ Lead aprons or thyroid shields should be used when appropriate.[13]

○ Personal monitoring devices may need to be worn by staff if the 'weekly workload exceeds 100 intra-oral or 50 panoramic films.'[14]

Film badges

The most commonly used type of personal monitoring device consists of an outer plastic case with a variety of windows of different thicknesses of plastic and three metal filters. A wrapped film is contained within the case, which is worn at hip level as a badge for a month, after which time the film is developed (see Figure 5.2). Any exposure to radiation will result in some degree of blackening on the film. The exact pattern of blackening seen on the film will depend on the energy of the beam and its penetrating ability.

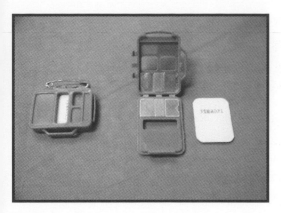

Figure 5.2: Left: film badge containing film ready to wear; right: film badge open and displayng plastic filters, open window and metal filters.

Clinical governance

Clinical governance demands that standards are established and met and that a clinical audit is carried out to ensure that this is the case. Risk assessment needs to be carried out in order to ensure the safest possible working environment for staff and to ensure that patients undergo procedures with minimal risk. Strict adherence to legislation such as IR(ME)R 2000 and working within guidelines such as those produced by the NRPB for Dental Practitioners as well as observance of local rules should ensure compliance with clinical governance.

Legislation

The following legislation applies to any person involved in any aspect of X-ray production such as dental nurses who are involved in the processing of X-ray films.

Dental nurses are not allowed to take X-rays unless they hold a qualification in dental radiography for dental nurses.

The IR(ME)R 2000[15] supersede the Protection of Persons Undergoing Medical Examination or Treatment Regulations (POPUMET) and became law on 13 May 2000.[16] This document defines the roles of operators, practitioners and referrers and the requirements for justifying and making an exposure. Under IR(ME)R 2000 the employer must provide written procedures for all medical exposures and an equipment inventory must be kept. Quality assurance and clinical audit are essential parts of the process in order to keep the dose to the patient as low as reasonably practicable. Equipment must be maintained regularly and records kept of any maintenance carried out.

Principles of dental radiography

Familiarity with the different techniques used will help the dental nurse decide which films and holders the operator will require in order to undertake the examination. (DN14.1)

X-ray film

There are two different types of film:

○ Direct action film is used to form images by X-rays (e.g. periapicals, bitewings, occlusals).

○ Indirect action film is used to form images by light emitted from the intensifying screens inside the cassette holding the film (e.g. dental panoramics, bimolars, lateral cephalometric skulls).

Films may be of different speeds and the fastest suitable film speed should be used in order to minimise patient dose. When using indirect action film, care must be taken to select a safe light with the correct spectral emission for the film used, for example a red safe light can be used for green and blue sensitive film.

Digital imaging

This is a method of recording the image without using a film and either a direct or indirect method may be used. Both systems use conventional X-ray equipment. The direct method uses a reusable sensor instead of an X-ray film. This is known as a CCD or Charged Coupling Device and resembles a paralleling technique film holder. It cannot be autoclaved or cold sterilised and must be contained within a disposable plastic cover before being placed in the mouth (DN14.1). Once the exposure has been made, the data is fed directly from the sensor into the computer and the image can be viewed directly on a computer screen. The indirect method uses a re-usable phosphor plate instead of the X-ray film. This is placed inside a plastic envelope for hygienic reasons, as it cannot be autoclaved, once this is done it is placed in a conventional film holder (DN14.1). After the exposure is made the phosphor plate is mounted on a support and placed in a special drum-shaped computer scanner. The phosphor plate is scanned, the data is fed into a computer from the scanner and the image is displayed on a computer monitor screen. Before being re-used the image must be removed from the phosphor plate by exposure to very bright light for a few minutes, such as that produced by a viewing box.

These methods have several advantages over conventional radiography:

○ Images can be manipulated and enhanced.

○ Images can be rejected due to exposure error and can be improved upon, thus minimising the need to repeat the procedure.

○ Processing errors can be eliminated.

○ It is claimed that the dose to the patient is lower than in conventional radiography.

○ Films can be stored on disc.

○ Films can be transferred electronically, thus minimising the risk of their being lost in the post.

Disadvantages include:

○ Initially quite a high investment is required.

○ Data must be securely stored.

○ Data must be backed up.

○ Hard copies can be obtained, but good quality thermal printers are expensive and there is some loss of resolution.

Intra-oral radiography

This type of radiography covers procedures where the film is placed inside the patient's mouth (for example using bitewings, periapicals and occlusals). In intra-oral radiography the image is formed as a direct result of X-rays sensitising the film, but these films are still sensitive to light and are protected from light fogging with a waterproof and light-proof film packet, which should only be removed in darkroom conditions. Inside the film packet the film is wrapped in black paper to prevent light leakage should the integrity of the outer wrapper be damaged and also to protect the film from physical damage. To prevent back scatter each package contains lead foil, which is placed behind the film between the black paper and the outer wrapper. Some film packets are contained within an extra polythene outer wrapper, which is discarded as soon as the film is taken, to prevent cross infection.

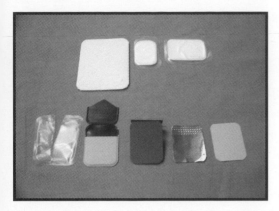

Figure 5.3: Top row: different sizes of intra-oral film, bottom row: contents of intra-oral film packet.

Periapicals

As its name suggests this type of radiography occurs when the apex of the tooth and surrounding bone needs to be visualised and selection criteria commonly include periapical pathology, root morphology, retained roots, trauma, endodontic treatment and periodontal disease. There are two distinctly different techniques that may be employed:

(a) Paralleling technique is the preferred method, because it is considered to produce the least distorted image, enables standardisation and offers increased reproducibility. It is considered to be the best view for assessing tooth-length and bone levels and is also preferred because the method used avoids unnecessary exposure of the patient's fingers.[17] The film is placed in a film holder behind the tooth so that it is parallel to the long axis of the tooth. In order to ensure that the long axis of the film and the tooth are as parallel as possible it is necessary to place the film some distance from the tooth and therefore, in order to prevent magnification of the image, it is essential that a collimator measuring 200 mm is used.[18] The film holder is connected to an indicator rod and localising ring. The central ray is directed parallel to the indicator rod and the open end of the collimator is aligned with the localising ring so that the central ray is centred to the tooth and to the film. Some patients with very small mouths, extreme gag reflexes or limited opening are unable to tolerate film holders.

(b) Bisecting angle technique is useful when patients cannot tolerate film holders or where a fracture is suspected, since the oblique rays used in this view exaggerate fracture lines. The film is placed in close proximity behind the tooth. Although film holders are available, they are difficult to use and the film is usually supported using the patient's finger or artery forceps. The central ray is directed perpendicular to the line bisecting the long axis of the tooth and the film and is centred to the apex of the tooth. This view is difficult to reproduce as it is dependent on the skill of the operator in assessing the exact angulation required. Since this

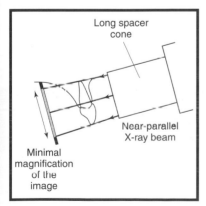

Figure 5.4: The theory of paralleling technique.

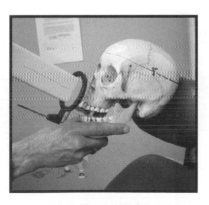

Figure 5.5: The correct placement of the X-ray film, holder and collimator.

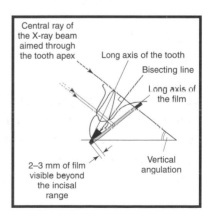

Figure 5.6: Theory of bisecting angle technique.

projection gives an oblique view of the crown it is difficult to assess depth of caries and films are more likely to be foreshortened or elongated than when the paralleling technique is used.

Bitewings

This view is taken to demonstrate the crowns and biting surfaces of the upper and lower teeth and interstitial spaces. They are usually taken with the long axis of the film horizontal but may be taken with the long axis vertical to demonstrate periodontal disease in adults or developing permanent dentition in children. The use of film holders, beam aiming devices and rectangular collimation is recommended.

Occlusals

The most common occlusal view is the upper anterior occlusal, which is taken to show the pathology of the anterior part of the maxilla and demonstrates the presence of unerupted teeth. The film is placed flat in the mouth and the beam is angled about 60 degrees downwards. Other types of occlusal view include the upper standard occlusal, which uses a steeper angulation and lower occlusals, which may be taken with the beam at 90 degrees to the part under examination to demonstrate the true position of unerupted teeth or oblique occlusals to demonstrate salivary stones. Both upper and lower occlusal views can be modified to provide a view similar to a bisecting angle periapical film to show anterior teeth in young children.

Extra-oral radiography

This covers views in which the film is placed outside the patient's mouth (e.g. dental panoramics, bimolars, lateral cephalometric skulls and occipto-mental sinus projection). Extra-oral views are taken using special films designed to be sensitive to a certain wavelength of light as well as to X-rays. The film is contained within a cassette to protect it from the light. Both front and back covers of the cassette are lined with intensifying screens that contain crystals that fluoresce (i.e. emit light of the specified wavelength when they are exposed to X-rays). This process intensifies the effect of the X-rays on the film and enables us to reduce patient exposure. If intensifying screens are to be used, care must be taken when selecting the colour of the safe lights as the spectral emission of the safe light must not be the same wavelength as the spectral sensitivity of the film. If the wavelengths are the same light fogging will occur.

Preparation of equipment (DN14.1)

The posterior and anterior film holders used for intra-oral techniques must be assembled correctly prior to use and care should be taken that, once the indicator rod is connected to the biteblock and the localising device is in place, the biteblock is centrally placed within the localising device. Assembled film holders and the correct number of unexposed films must be placed white side up on a clean denta-nap or paper towel and exposed films should be placed coloured side up so that there can be no confusion between the two, in order to avoid accidental double exposure. After the examination is complete the film holder assembly should be dismantled prior to being sterilised.

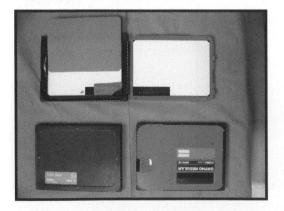

Figure 5.7: Film cassettes.

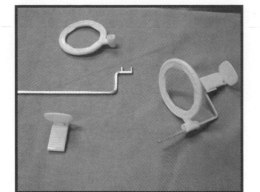

Figure 5.8:
Posterior
holder.

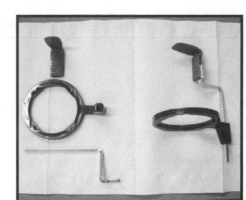

Figure 5.9:
Anterior
holder.

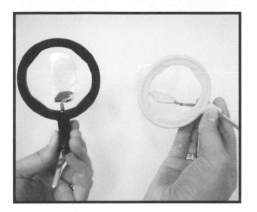

Figure 5.10:
Assembled
posterior
and anterior
holders.

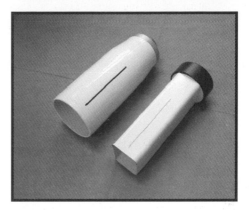

Figure 5.11:
Collimators.

Preparation of patients (DN14.1)

○ The patient's identity must be checked.

○ The patient should be asked about any possibility of pregnancy although as already discussed this is not usually a contra-indication for dental radiography.

○ The patient should be asked to remove all radio-opaque objects from around the head and neck prior to a DPT being taken.

○ A brief explanation of the procedure and clear instructions should be given to the patient prior to the commencement of the examination in order to eliminate the need to repeat the X-ray.

QUESTIONS

Question 1

Write a brief summary of the protocol in your practice showing how you would take into consideration any special needs each patient may have.

Cross infection control for dental radiography (DN14.1)
☞

Intra-oral radiography

1. Gloves must be worn for the examination. After the examination these must be discarded in the yellow clinical waste bags.

2. Where possible, barrier-wrapped film should be used.

3. The exact number of films for each examination should be taken out of the box before the examination begins.

4. Exposed films should be placed coloured side up on a paper towel. At the end of the examination the barrier wrapping is removed and the unwrapped film, still in its light-proof cover, is dropped onto a clean surface. It is considered safe to place this in the hatch for the darkroom technician to process. If non-barrier wrapped film is used for any reason, extra precautions must be taken to ensure that contamination does not occur as the film is not 'clean'.

5. Used biteblocks, localising devices and indicator rods must be disconnected before sterilisation.

6. Once the examination is finished the X-ray tube and surfaces should be cleaned with an azowipe. Please note the equipment should be switched off in order to do this.

Extra-orals

1. Although gloves are not always necessary for all extra-oral examinations, in some cases, such as for dental panoramic radiographs, it may be appropriate to wear gloves in order to assist the patient to locate the groove on the bite-block with their front teeth. If gloves are used they should be discarded in the yellow clinical waste bins.

2. Any equipment that comes into direct contact with the patient during the examination, such as chin rest, temporal supports, ear-pieces and cassettes (e.g. during a bimolar examination), should be cleaned with alcohol once the examination is finished. Equipment should be switched off in order to do this to eliminate risk of electric shock.

3. Biteblocks must be sterilised if they are to be re-used.

?

QUESTIONS

Question 2

Summarise the cross infection protocols for (a) intra-oral radiography and (b) extra-oral radiography in your workplace.

_____

_____

_____

_____

Film processing and darkroom practice
☞

X-Ray films contain silver halide crystals such as silver bromide suspended in a gelatin emulsion. The black and white appearance of the processed radiograph results from either the presence or absence of black metallic silver in the emulsion. The black areas indicate that the crystals have been exposed and the clear areas are unexposed. Processing is the means by which the latent (hidden image) in the exposed radiograph is revealed and made permanent. Care must be taken when handling the film before and after exposure. Films damaged before exposure bear white marks, whereas those damaged after exposure will bear a dark mark (DN14.2). Films should be stored in a cool dry place, away from chemicals, ionising radiation and direct sunlight. Stock must be strictly controlled to monitor expiry dates and should be rotated to ensure that the oldest films are used first. The rate of film usage should be monitored so that sufficient film is ordered to cope with the demand of your practice.

Chemicals must be mixed in well-ventilated areas according to the manufacturer's instructions. The solutions must be maintained at optimum temperature and the temperature of the solution should be checked prior to usage. Chemicals need to be replenished regularly and exhausted or discoloured chemicals should be replaced.

Constituents and action of developer and fixer

Developer	Fixer
Reducing agents convert silver halide crystals to black metallic silver and free bromide	Fixing agents convert unexposed silver halide crystals into a soluble form
Alkali – buffer	Acetic acid – buffer
Preservative e.g. potassium sulphite	Preservative e.g. potassium sulphite
Restrainer e.g. potassium bromide[19]	Hardener (aluminium sulphate)
Lubricant (glycol)	Solvent – water
Solvent – water	

Comparison of stages in different methods of processing

☞ It is essential that all stages of film processing are carried out in the correct order – time and temperature are critical.

Automatic processing	Standard processing	Rapid manual processing (special chemicals)
Film is unwrapped in safe light conditions	Film is unwrapped in safe light conditions	Film is unwrapped in safe light conditions
Film is fed into the processor under safe light conditions and enters the developer	Film is developed in dark or safe light conditions for 4 minutes at 21°C	Film is developed in the dark or or under safe light conditions for 1 minute at room temperature
Film passes through squeegee rollers that remove any excess developer before passing into the fixer tank	Film is washed[20] thoroughly to remove excess developer	Film is washed thoroughly to remove excess developer
Film passes through squeegee rollers to remove excess fixer	Film is fixed (clearing time[21] plus ten minutes)	Film is fixed for two minutes
Film passes through the wash tank	Film is washed for twenty minutes	Film is washed for several minutes in running water
Film passes through squeegee rollers to remove excess water and then passes into dryer	Film is either dried in a drying cabinet or left overnight to dry.[22]	Film is either dried in a drying cabinet or left overnight to dry

☞

Inadequate washing may result in the by-products of processing being retained within the emulsion and some discolouration of the image may occur. Care must be taken to ensure that films are completely dry prior to mounting otherwise mould can form on the surface of the emulsion.

Safe lights

Must conform to the following specifications:

○ 25 watt bulb

○ Appropriately coloured filter (regularly inspected for cracks)

○ Minimum of 1.25M (4 feet) above the work surface.

The 'safe' film handling time can be determined with a coin test. A strip of numbered coins is placed across the film in safe light conditions and covered with a card. The card is slowly pulled across the coins so that for each 10-second period another coin is exposed to the safe light. The film is processed and the maximum 'safe' handling time can easily be calculated by noting which number coin has caused an outline on the film and multiplying the number by 10 seconds. Failure to process a film within the 'safe' handling time will result in fogging.

QUESTIONS

Question 3

Carry out a coin test to determine the safe handling time for the darkroom in your practice.

_____

_____

_____

_____

Common faults caused by poor darkroom practice (DN14.2 AND DN14.3)

Fault	Usual cause
Film completely black	White light fogging
No image on film	Either (a) no exposure has been made, or (b) there was no developer in the tank, or (c) the film was outside the field of radiation
White crimp marks on film	Manhandling before exposure
Black crimp marks on film	Manhandling after exposure
Green or pink opaque film	Processing has not occurred
Sepia effect	Inadequate fixing or inadequate washing
Dichroic fog[23]	If fixer has contaminated the developer
Pye marks	Scratches due to debris on the rollers
Static marks	Due to nylon clothing or other synthetic fabrics worn by operator
Staining	Due to splashes of chemicals or films being caught up in the rollers and jammed in the developer tank for a prolonged period
Dark and grainy film	Excessive development time or too high a temperature
Pale films	Exhausted chemicals, insufficient development time or too low a temperature

Miscellaneous faults

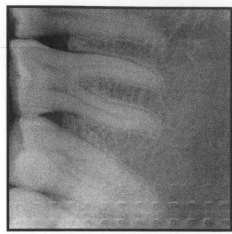

Figure 5.12:
An X-ray image.

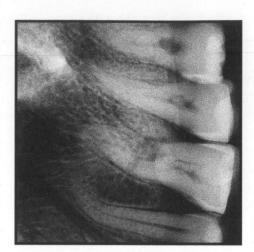

Figure 5.13:
An X-ray image.

Film was placed back to front in the holder and so the image of the lead foil was projected over the lower 2nd and 3rd molars. The film appears pale because lead has attenuated some of the radiation. It is correctly mounted in this instance if the dot is placed upside down.

Rough handling by the operator, when removing the film from the holder, has resulted in crimp marks. These run diagonally across the root of the upper first premolar to the top of the film.

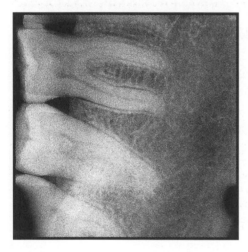

Figure 5.14:
An X-ray image.

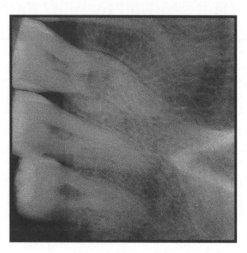

Figure 5.15:
An X-ray image.

The envelope was partly open and light has leaked in and caused partial fogging. This can be seen over the crown of the lower third molar and along the bottom edge of the film.

The film was manually processed. The temperature of the chemicals was too low and to compensate for this the film has been left in the developer too long, which has resulted in poor contrast and a grainy appearance. There is a scratch on the surface of the film caused by the forceps used for supporting the film in the chemicals.

Film mounting (DN14.2)

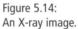

Films must be securely mounted, the right way round, dated and accurately labelled with the patient's name and number for archiving in the patient's notes. Extra-oral films should have an anatomical marker denoting which is the right side and which is the left. Intra-oral films are marked with an embossed dot that serves as an anatomical marker. If the convex (raised) side of the dot is facing you then the film is the correct way round. The tooth can then be identified using anatomical landmarks and root morphology.

Features of the maxilla and teeth	Features of the mandible and teeth
The bony trabeculae (pattern) are often more tightly woven in the upper jaw and the vertical striations are more pronounced	The bony trabeculae are often more loosely woven in the lower jaw and the horizontal striations are more pronounced
The upper incisor and canine teeth are larger than the lowers	The lower incisor and canine teeth are often smaller than the uppers
In the premolar and molar region the maxillary sinus can be seen just above the roots of the teeth	In the molar region the inferior dental nerve can be seen running like two parallel lines just below the roots of the teeth
Upper molars usually have three roots	Lower molars usually have two roots
The roots of upper molars are usually bunched together as if they are trying to hang on	The roots of lower molars are usually spread apart as if they are trying to balance standing up

Quality assurance and film fault analysis (DN14.1)

Under IR(ME)R 2000, the employer must provide written procedures for all medical exposure and an equipment inventory must be kept. Quality assurance of standard operating procedures and clinical audit are an essential part of the process in order to keep the dose to the patient as low as reasonably practicable (this is called the ALARP principle).

Under IRR99 the employer must also establish quality assurance programmes for medical equipment. Quality assurance is an essential component of clinical governance, which involves setting a standard and monitoring the system being tested to ensure that standards are being met. Written records must be kept for each patient of the number of films taken and the exposure factors used.

The following types of quality assurance should be undertaken in the dental surgery:

○ Sensitometry, i.e. the processing of an image of a test object or step wedge for comparison to a control film must be carried out to monitor processor performance (DN14.3).

○ Check levels of chemicals and replenish if required (DN14.1).

○ Monitor and record temperature of processing chemicals (DN14.1).

○ Record of maintenance on processors and X-ray equipment (DN14.1).

○ Step wedge tests or the exposure of a test object to check output of X-ray unit (DN14.3).

○ Coin tests to check safe lights.

○ Film fault analysis (DN14.3).

○ Clinical audit (DN14.3).

Sensitometric strips can be produced either by exposing an X-ray film that is covered by a step wedge (a strip of metal with steps of graduated thickness), or with a sensitometer — a device that exposes an X-ray film to light of varying intensities to produce a film with a series of different degrees of blackening. The density or degree of blackness on the film can be measured with a special optical instrument called a densitometer and the difference in the reading between two steps gives an indication of the contrast. In the absence of sensitometric equipment or a step wedge some simple test tools can be made by filling a small plastic box with a variety of items such as blue tack, a screw, a tooth and a paperclip, alternatively a step wedge can be constructed by wrapping different thicknesses of lead foil around a tongue depressor. The test tool is placed over an X-ray film and an exposure is made. The processed image can be compared with a control image and any visual difference will indicate a problem with the system. It is essential that the same distance and exposure factors are used each time the test tool is used and that these are recorded.

QUESTIONS

?

Question 4

Describe the procedure in your workplace for testing the image quality and the process for reporting failure of the equipment to comply with the required standard.

Film fault analysis and audit

The NRPB recommends that a numerical system is used to denote the grading of each film taken. Grade 1 film is excellent and 70 per cent of films should fall into this category, Grade 2 is diagnostically acceptable and Grade 3 unacceptable and fewer than 10 per cent of films should fall into this category.[24] All Grade 3 films are considered to be rejects and should be analysed to minimise errors (DN14.3).

☞ Common film fault categories include:

○ Exposure – films may be too light if underexposed or too dark if overexposed.

○ Positioning faults include – **(a)** periapical films with missing crown or apices.

　　　　　　　　　　　　　　　(b) elongated or foreshortened teeth due to incorrect angulation.

　　　　　　　　　　　　　　　(c) bitewings with enamel edges overlapping.

○ Darkroom – as discussed previously (DN14.3).

○ Movement – patient movement results in a blurred image and interrupted outline to structures.

○ Miscellaneous fault.[25]

The data from film fault analysis must be recorded and it may be helpful to plot graphs each month so that progress can be monitored.

Records must be kept of each exposure made for each patient and the number of films taken and the exposure factors used. Radiographs must be correctly and securely mounted and clearly labelled and stored so that they can be traced easily (DN14.2).

☞ Audits should be carried out periodically to ensure that this is being done.

QUESTIONS

Question 5

Describe the audit process in your workplace.

_____

_____

_____

_____

Health and safety and risk assessment

☞ Risk assessments are essential components of clinical governance and are vital in maintaining a safe environment for staff, patients and others. All potential hazards and the degree of severity of the harm they could cause as well as the likelihood of the harm occurring need to be considered and precautions must be introduced to eliminate risk of harm to staff, patients and others.

In the surgery

☞ Hazards in a surgery where X-rays are to be taken include:

○ Risk of unnecessary exposure of staff, patients or relatives to radiation

○ Risk of electric shock

○ Risk of cross infection

○ Risk of muscular-skeletal injury when handling patients or equipment.

In order to eliminate risk of unnecessary exposure of staff, patients or relatives to radiation, local rules and employer's protocols must be provided and strictly adhered to by all personnel. Staff may be required to wear radiation monitoring devices if the 'weekly workload is in excess of 100 intra-oral or 50 panoramic films.'[26]

Question 6

List the measures in place in your workplace to protect (a) staff, (b) patients and (c) others.

_____

_____

_____

_____

_____

_____

Film processors and X-ray units must be regularly maintained (DN14.1) and a quality assurance programme must be in place to ensure that equipment is safe to operate and to monitor the performance of all equipment. X-ray equipment must not be operated with wet hands and should be isolated from the mains when it is being cleaned.

Cross-infection control measures should be in place to protect patients and operators and should include the use of barrier-wrapped films and gloves. Equipment and surfaces should be cleaned between patients and must be kept free of dust and dirt. (DN14.1)

In order to eliminate risk of muscular-skeletal injury, lifting and handling protocols should be in place and staff should be trained in patient handling techniques and must consider the ergonomics of their working environment prior to moving patients or equipment.

In the darkroom

Hazards in the darkroom include:

○   Working in the dark

○   Handling chemicals

○   Risk of electric shock

○   Risk of cross infection

○   Risk of injury from moving machine parts

○   Intrusion during processing resulting in accidental exposure of the film to white light.

Care should be taken to eliminate the risk of tripping over objects in the dark and unnecessary furniture should be removed from the area. Essential furniture should be marked with reflective strips to alert staff to its presence when the safe lights are on. The floor should be dry to eliminate the risk of slipping.

The Control of Substances Hazardous to Health Regulations 1994 (COSSH) require all potentially harmful substances to be identified and under these regulations employers are required to undertake risk assessments and introduce measures to control or eliminate exposure to all hazardous substances. Processing chemicals must be stored safely and prepared in well-ventilated conditions (DN14.1). The level of chemicals in the machine must be checked and replenished regularly, discoloured or exhausted chemicals should be replaced (DN14.2). The chemicals must be made up correctly according to the manufacturer's instructions in order to ensure that they are of the correct concentration and they must be maintained at the correct temperature for optimum working conditions (DN14.2). Goggles, masks and waterproof gloves must be worn when chemicals are being handled or when routine processor maintenance is being carried out. Chemicals must be handled carefully to ensure that one solution does not contaminate another and separate utensils should be used for fixer and developer (DN14.2). Any spills should be cleaned up immediately. Waste chemicals must be disposed of safely and in accordance with local regulations, silver must be recovered from used fixer prior to disposal (DN14.3). Silver recovery units are available and some companies dealing in disposal of waste chemicals also provide a silver recovery service.

To safeguard staff against electric shocks, processors must be kept in good working order and should be checked for electrical safety. Care must be taken when using electrical equipment that hands are dry.

Cross-infection control measures must be introduced to avoid contamination of work surfaces. Working surfaces must be kept dust free (DN14.1). Barrier-wrapped films should be used for intra-oral films and should not be taken into the darkroom area until the contaminated outer covers have been removed.

Long hair should be tied back and staff should secure loose items of clothing, such as scarves or ties, to minimise the risk of hair or clothing being caught in the entry rollers of the processor.

In the absence of a light-proof maze entrance to the darkroom or revolving doors, the darkroom door should be lockable to prevent intrusion during processing and safeguard against accidental exposure of the X-ray film to white light. Film hoppers should be fitted with micro-switches so that white light cannot accidentally be switched on should the hopper be open (DN14.2).

References

[1] This certificate was jointly approved by the Dental Nurses Standards and Training Advisory Board and the College of Radiographers in 1991, The College of Radiographers, *Dental Radiography Course for Dental Surgery Assistants*, (London, The College of Radiographers, 1994).

[2] Ball, J.L. and Moore, A.D., *Essential Physics for Radiographers*, (Oxford, London, Edinburgh, Blackwell Scientific Publications, 1980), 159.

[3] Whaites, E., *Essentials of Dental Radiography and Radiology*, (Edinburgh, Harcourt Publishers, 2002), 29.

[4] Whaites, E., *Essentials of Dental Radiography and Radiology*, (Edinburgh, Harcourt Publishers, 2002), 29.

[5] Mason refers to the prevalence of ulcerative dermatitis on the hands of operators in the absence of proper protective measures when radiography was in its infancy. Mason, R., *A Guide to Dental Radiography*, (Bristol, John Wright & Sons Ltd.), 1 & 2.

[6] Whaites highlights the particular hazard associated with Radon gas, a natural decay product of uranium in some areas including parts of Cornwall and Scotland where the ground rock is granite. The gas permeates the soil and infiltrates houses. Whaites, E., *Essentials of Dental Radiography and Radiology*, (Edinburgh, Harcourt Publishers, 2002), 26.

[7] Levinson has emphasised that 'On no account must a nurse hold the film in place for a patient; if a child cannot keep it still, the parent must hold it in place.' Levinson, H., *Textbook for Dental Nurses*, (Oxford, Blackwell Sciences Ltd, 1997), 395. N.B. The adult holding the child should not be pregnant.

[8] NRPB, *Guidance Notes for Dental Practitioners on the Safe Use of X-Ray Equipment*, (National Radiological Protection Board, June 2001), 20.

[9] Films or detectors should only be supported by the patient if an appropriate holder cannot be tolerated by the patient. Ibid, 25.

[10] This is sometimes referred to as the ALARP principle.

[11] NRPB, *Guidance Notes for Dental Practitioners on the Safe Use of X-Ray Equipment*, (National Radiological Protection Board, June 2001), 28.

[12] Although on the whole in dental radiography the primary beam does not pass through the pelvis, the NRPB recommends that 'due to the emotive nature of radiography during pregnancy, the patient could be given the option of delaying the radiography'. NRPB, *Guidance Notes for Dental Practitioners on the Safe Use of X-Ray Equipment*, (National Radiological Protection Board, June 2001), 14. **N.B.** This is particularly valid if treatment is to be delayed due to pregnancy, as a current radiograph immediately prior to treatment is usually required.

[13] The NRPB does not recommend that lead aprons are used routinely for dental radiography, but suggests that they may be used if the patient is pregnant and that thyroid collars should be used only if the thyroid is in the primary beam. NRPB, *Guidance Notes for Dental Practitioners on the Safe Use of X-Ray Equipment*, (National Radiological Protection Board, June 2001), 26

[14] Ibid, 19

[15] The Ionising Radiation (Medical Exposure) Regulations 2000

[16] IR(ME)R 2000

[17] The NRPB guidelines recommend the usage of film holders, beam aiming devices and rectangular collimation not exceeding 40 x 50 mm in the taking of periapical films. NRPB, *Guidance Notes for Dental Practitioners on the Safe Use of X-Ray Equipment*, (National Radiological Protection Board, June 2001), 29

[18] The NRPB guidelines recommend the usage of film holders, beam aiming devices and rectangular collimation not exceeding 40 x 50 mm in the taking of periapical films. NRPB, *Guidance Notes for Dental Practitioners on the Safe Use of X-Ray Equipment*, (National Radiological Protection Board, June 2001), 29. Historically, dental collimators were shorter than this and the need for a longer collimator led to this technique being dubbed 'the long cone technique'.

[19] Restrainer helps to prevent chemical fogging and is only added to newly made-up solutions since bromine is produced as a waste product during development and will build up in the solution with time. For this reason it is sometimes referred to as 'Starter solution' (DN14.2, point 4).

[20] Either running water or an 'acid stop bath' should be used. Since developer works best in alkaline conditions the acid stop bath has the advantage of immediately stopping any further action of the developer as well as rinsing off excess chemicals.

[21] Clearing time is the amount of time in seconds that it takes for the film to lose its cloudy appearance and become transparent. This can be visualised because once the film has been placed into the fixer it is safe to expose the film to white light. Inadequately fixed films become sepia tinted (yellow) with time and deteriorate.

[22] Films should not be left in the water for long periods i.e. overnight as the emulsion may start to dissolve.

[23] Dichroic means two colours. This fault occurs when developer is contaminated by fixer, during routine processor maintenance or splashing from the chemical tanks. There is usually a characteristic odour of ammonia.

[24] NRPB, *Guidance Notes for Dental Practitioners on the Safe Use of X-Ray Equipment*, (National Radiological Protection Board, June 2001), 33

[25] These can include just about anything as the name suggests, but strict adherence of the operator to protocols and clear instructions to the patients should help to keep these faults and others to a minimum

[26] NRPB, *Guidance Notes for Dental Practitioners on the Safe Use of X-Ray Equipment*, (National Radiological Protection Board, June 2001), 19

ORAL HEALTH AND THE PREVENTION OF PERIODONTAL DISEASE AND DENTAL CARIES

6

Introduction

This chapter is linked to DN15.1 of the NVQ Level 3 in Oral Health Care. Two of the most common diseases in the world are dental caries and periodontal disease. This chapter will look at the factors involved in causing these diseases, how they may be treated and, most importantly, prevented.

It will also look at the role of the dental nurse (DN) in connection with the preparation of clinical environments, chairside support and oral health education. First, the anatomy of the tooth and periodontium will be discussed to aid understanding of the effect each disease has on the oral and dental tissues.

SECTION 1: Anatomy of the tooth and periodontium

The tooth comprises the crown, which is visible in the oral cavity and the root, which is embedded within the bone of the jaws, and is not normally visible. The main parts of a tooth are the enamel, dentine and pulp. The tooth is supported within the alveolar bone of the upper maxilla and lower mandible by ligaments and a cement-like substance covering the root called cementum. The alveolar bone is covered by a tissue known as the gingiva, which also acts as a support structure to the tooth (Figure 6.1).

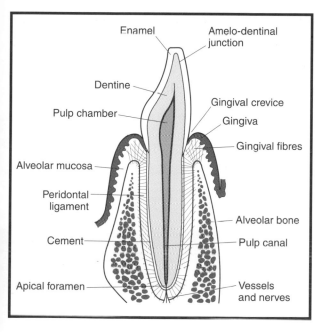

Figure 6.1: Cross section of a single-rooted tooth.

Enamel

The outer covering of the crown is made up of a mineral called enamel, which is whitish in colour and is the hardest substance in the body. If viewed under the microscope, millions of interlocking crystals made up of a material similar to a substance known as hydroxyapatite can be seen.

☞ Chemically, hydroxyapatite is built up of calcium and phosphate ions, and it is these ions that are lost during demineralisation caused by dental caries. The crystals run from the inner to the outer surface of enamel and are known as enamel rods or prisms. Although these crystals are hard they are susceptible to being dissolved by acid. Enamel does not contain nerves or blood vessels and therefore is insensitive to pain.

Dentine

The next layer of the tooth is made up of a partially mineralised substance known as dentine, which lies under the enamel of the crown and also forms the outer surface of the root. Dentine is yellowish in colour and is also made up of crystals of hydroxyapatite, but in smaller concentrations than enamel. Dentine is softer than enamel but harder than bone. When viewed under a microscope, thousands of small channels, known as dentinal tubules, can be seen running from the inner surface of the dentine to the junction with the enamel. These tubules contain cell processes, which come from cells lining the pulp chamber, called odontoblasts. Odontoblasts continue to lay down new dentine throughout the life of the tooth, and they also lay down more dentine in response to a stimulus such as dental caries. This helps to protect the pulp from damage and keep the tooth alive. Unlike enamel, dentine can feel the sensation of pain due to its connection with the pulp.

Pulp

The pulp chamber and canals lie under the dentine and contain a soft tissue that consists of blood vessels, lymphatic vessels and nerves, which keep the tooth alive. As mentioned in the previous section, odontoblasts, which line the pulpal walls, continue to produce dentine throughout life; this has the effect of making the pulp chamber and canals smaller over time. The pulp feels pain and can become infected, which may then lead to pulp death and death of the tooth. The nerves and blood vessels leave the pulp canal via a small hole or foramen located at the apex of the root (Figure 6.2).

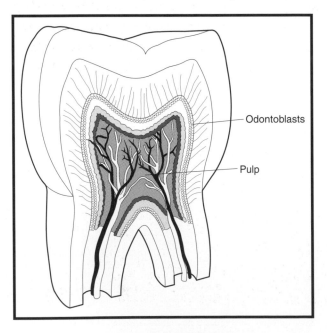

Figure 6.2: Cross section of a multi-rooted tooth.

The periodontium

The periodontium is the support structure of the teeth and it consists of the following four components (Figure 6.3).

○   The gingivae

○   The alveolar bone

○   The periodontal ligament

○   The cementum.

The gingiva

The gingiva covers the alveolar bone and forms part of the support structure of the tooth. There are two main parts to the gingiva, the marginal gingival (also known as the free gingiva), which forms a cuff about 1–2 mm wide around the neck of the tooth, and the attached gingiva, which is connected to the underlying alveolar bone. The marginal gingival can be pulled away from the side of the tooth with a probe, as it is not attached to any underlying structure, (hence the name free gingiva). The gap between the tooth and the marginal gingiva is known as the gingival sulcus, and in health can be between 0–2 mm in depth. The attached gingiva, when healthy, is pink in colour (with variations for ethnicity) and its surface appears to be stippled. The gingiva in-between the teeth is known as the interdental papilla.

The alveolar bone

The alveolar bone makes up the bone in the socket in the upper jaw (maxilla) and the lower jaw (mandible). Alveolar bone consists of two main layers: compact bone and spongy or cancellous bone. The compact bone is found on the buccal and lingual surfaces of the jaws and also lining the socket. The compact bone of the socket is slightly different from that on the outer surfaces as it consists of many tiny holes, which allow access of blood vessels to the tooth. It is important that bone has a good blood supply because it is a dynamic structure that is constantly changing and remodelling.

The periodontal ligament

The periodontal ligament connects the tooth to the alveolar bone and consists of many collagen fibres (see Figure 6.4). These fibres generally run from the cementum on the root of the tooth to the alveolar bone. The periodontal ligament also contains blood vessels, lymphatic vessels and nerves. It is interesting to note that the nerves of the pulp can only transmit pain impulses to the brain, whilst

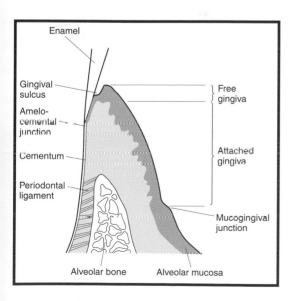

Figure 6.3: The periodontium.

those of the periodontal ligament also transmit sensations of light touch and pressure. The periodontal ligament supports the tooth in the socket and acts as a kind of 'shock absorber' so that when pressure is applied to the tooth, for example when biting down, it allows the tooth to move a fraction in the socket. If a tooth were stuck rigid in alveolar bone it would probably crack under the stress of biting. The periodontal ligament is divided into a number of groups depending on their position of attachment. The groups include:

○ Alveolar crest fibres – which run from the cementum, on the neck of the tooth, in a downwards direction to the alveolar crest.

○ Horizontal fibres – which run horizontally from the cementum to the alveolar crest.

○ Oblique fibres – which run in an apical direction from the alveolar bone and insert into the cementum on the main part of the root.

○ Apical fibres – run from the cementum, on the apex of the tooth, to the base of the socket.

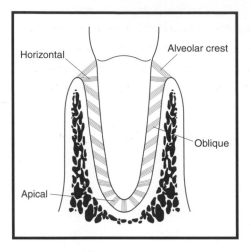

Figure 6.4: Periodontal ligament fibres.

Cementum

Cementum covers the root of the tooth and is yellowish in colour. Approximately half of its structure is mineralised with hydroxyapatite, the other half consisting of an organic material and water. The cementum is an important support structure of the tooth, because it is one half of the attachment for the periodontal ligament that holds the tooth in the alveolar bone.

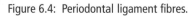

SECTION 2: Dental caries linked to DN19.1

Introduction

This section will cover:

○ The cause of dental caries
○ The spread of dental caries through the dental tissues
○ Diagnosis of dental caries
○ Prevention of dental caries.

Dental caries is a disease of the mineralised tissues of the teeth, namely:

○ enamel
○ dentine
○ cementum.

Dental caries is caused when the bacteria in plaque convert certain sugars in the diet into acid. This acid will demineralise the mineral portion of the tooth (enamel, part of the dentine and cementum) and then break down the organic part (rest of the dentine, cementum and pulp).

The cause of dental caries

Certain types of bacteria in plaque are able to convert fermentable carbohydrates in the diet (e.g. foods containing the sugars such as sucrose and fructose) into acid. The acid will make the pH of plaque fall below 5.5 within one to three minutes. Repeated falls in pH over time may result in the demineralisation of the tooth surface, resulting in breakdown of the enamel surface, and eventually creating a cavity.

Dental plaque (DN19.1 and DN19.2)

Dental plaque is a soft, non-calcified bacterial deposit that accumulates on the surfaces of the teeth and other objects in the mouth, such as dentures, bridges and restorations. It adheres strongly and can only be removed effectively by mechanical means such as brushing. It is composed of 70 per cent bacteria and 30 per cent interbacterial substances, including food debris, epithelial cells and erythrocytes (Red cells). After the tooth surface has been cleaned it quickly becomes coated with an organic film called the pellicle, which helps to attract bacteria to the tooth surface.

☞ The important bacteria as far as dental caries is concerned are *mutans streptococci* and *lactobacilli*, which quickly convert fermentable carbohydrates into acid.

Keyes concept

Certain factors coming together are necessary for caries to occur (see Figure 6.5). These are:

○ Bacteria found in plaque.

○ Susceptible site which is the surface on the tooth that attracts most plaque and is harder to clean. Sites include the enamel pits and fissures on the occlusal surfaces of pre-molars and molars, and the approximal surfaces just below the contact point.

○ Fermentable carbohydrate, known as the substrate and includes the sugars: sucrose, glucose, fructose, dextrose and maltose. Sucrose is the sugar that is most quickly converted into acid.

○ Time which is a key factor, because repeated falls in plaque pH to below 5.5 will cause demineralisation.

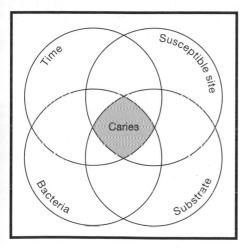

Figure 6.5: Keyes concept.

The Stephan Curve

The change in plaque pH may be represented graphically over a period of time following a glucose rinse. This graph is known as a Stephan Curve, after the person who first described it in 1944. As the graph shows, plaque pH can take up to 30–60 minutes to return to normal (Figure 6.6).

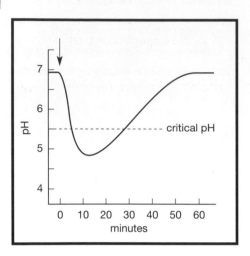

Figure 6.6: The Stephan Curve.

Demineralisation and remineralisation

If plaque pH repeatedly drops below 5.5 then demineralisation of the enamel will occur. During demineralisation calcium and phosphate ions are lost from the enamel structure. If enough time is allowed in-between falls in pH, saliva will help neutralise the acid and raise the pH, aiding remineralisation. Saliva also contains calcium and phosphate ions, and the enamel will absorb these.

☞ The remineralising benefits of saliva are improved when fluoride is present.

Diet and caries

The essential role of sugars in the diet causing dental caries has been established for some time. Evidence was collected from various studies that involved both humans and animals. Three human studies will now be highlighted.

Tristan da Cuhna

This is a remote rocky island in the south Atlantic whose inhabitants had an excellent dental state in the 1930s when their diet was confined to fish, meat and vegetables. However, after 1940 there was a sharp increase in the inhabitants' level of dental caries, which coincided with consumption of imported sugary foods.

Hopewood House

In 1942, an Australian businessman set up a children's home called Hopewood House for children from a low socio-economic background. He made sure that all the children were brought up on a healthy diet excluding all refined carbohydrates. Surveys of the time showed that the children all had a low experience of dental caries, compared with children of the same age and social background. However, when they left the home at 12 years old, and went back to a high refined carbohydrate diet, the caries rate was the same as other children of their age and social background. This showed that the diet of the children up to 12 years old gave them no protection from dental caries when returning to a high refined carbohydrate diet.

The Vipholm Study

This is a study that was carried out in a Swedish hospital for people with mental disabilities in the late 1930s and early 1940s. It was set up to look into the relationship between diet and dental caries, but it would not be allowed to be carried out today for ethical reasons.

The patients were divided into one control and six experimental groups. For one year all the patients received four meals a day that were relatively low in sugar, and no sugar was given between meals. During this time the number of new carious lesions was found to be very low. The following year dietary changes were made that involved the addition of large sucrose supplements in sticky or non-sticky form, either with or between meals. The effect on dental caries was then assessed.

The control group, who continued with the basic diet, showed little increase in caries throughout the study. In the experimental groups the diet was supplemented by:

- Sucrose drinks
- Sucrose in bread
- Chocolate
- Caramels
- 12 toffees per day
- 24 toffees per day.

There was a definite increase in caries in all groups except when the sucrose drink was taken at mealtimes. The highest risk of dental caries came from consuming sugar between meals, especially in a sticky form. In the 24-toffees per day group the increase in caries was so great when taken between meals, that the sugar supplement was withdrawn, which resulted in a fall in caries rate.

Sugars in the diet

Sugar is used as a flavouring and preservative, and is found in many popular foods and drinks. It is recommended that we consume less than **60g of refined sugar per day**, which is **12 teaspoons of sugar**, (dietary reference values of the COMA committee 1991), and recent studies estimate current daily consumption to be on average 95g. The sugars that are most responsible for causing dental caries are non-milk extrinsic sugars (NMES). These include sucrose and glucose that are added to foods and drinks during processing.

Spread of dental caries

Enamel

Plaque acids will break down the mineral component of enamel, causing demineralisation. The earliest clinical evidence of this will be the white spot lesion, which shows as a small white, opaque area on the enamel surface (see Figure 6.7). This area can be become brown due to is being porous and picking up stains. If no preventative measures are taken the lesion will become larger and caries will start to spread through the enamel towards the dentine.

Dentine and pulp

At the enamel–dentine junction caries will spread out to involve a larger area of the dentine underneath the enamel.The enamel will become undermined, leaving it unsupported, and it will eventually fracture and form a cavity.

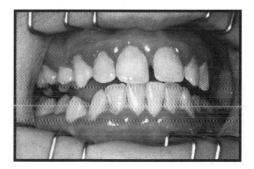

Figure 6.7: White and brown spot lesions.

Because the dentine is a living tissue, and is connected to the pulp by way of the odontoblastic processes in the dentinal tubules, it can defend itself from attack. Defence mechanisms include:

○ the tubules becoming blocked (tubular sclerosis) to try and prevent the caries progressing through the dentine

○ more dentine being laid down by the odontoblasts at the junction between the pulp and dentine, (reactionary dentine), to protect the pulp

○ inflammation of the pulp (pulpitis).

If no preventative measures are taken the caries will progress to the pulp, causing irrirvisible pulpitis and eventual death (necrosis) of the pulp. Infections from the pulp may tract out of the apex and cause an alveolar abscess.

Diagnosis of dental caries (DN15.1)

Early diagnosis of dental caries is important if it is to be prevented from spreading, and treated successfully. Patients who attend the dentist regularly will have more chance of the caries being picked up early, than those patients who only attend if they are in pain. Caries may be diagnosed in the following ways:

○ Observation – the dentist may notice that the enamel has a grey appearance, or there is an obvious cavitated lesion. White or brown spot lesions will be noted and monitored, and the patient given preventative advice.

○ Touch – The dentist may use straight/briault/sickle probes to feel gently around the surfaces of the teeth. Dental floss or tape, which will catch on carious lesion, may be used for the approximal areas.

○ Translumination – use of a fibre-optic light shows up caries as a dark shadow.

○ Radiographs – bitewings/periapicals/oblique laterals can be used to detect caries. A dark area of radiolucency will show where demineralisation has occurred. Bitewings are particularly effective at showing approximal caries.

○ Patient history – The patient may complain of sensitivity to hot/cold/sweet foods and drinks.

Treatment of dental caries (DN15.1 and DN15.2)

A more detailed description of the treatment of dental caries is covered in other chapters. However, the basic principles of treatment are prevention of pain, eradication of disease and restoration of function. This can be achieved by gaining access to the dental caries, removing it and restoring the tooth. A tooth may be at risk from secondary caries forming around and underneath the restoration if the patient is not given preventative advice and oral health education.

Prevention of dental caries

As dental caries is a multi-factorial disease, as illustrated by Keyes concept, many factors affect its prevention.

Diet (DN19.2)

Providing the patient with diet advice is vitally important in the prevention of dental caries. There are several areas that need to be covered including diet history, analysing a diet sheet and relevant preventative advice.

Diet history

The patient, or parents/guardians of a patient, will need their diet analysed, and one effective way of carrying this out is to complete a diet sheet (see Figure 6.8). At the initial visit a 24-hour diet history may be carried out. This involves asking the patient to recall everything they have eaten or drunk from the beginning of the previous day. From this information the frequency and amount of refined carbohydrates the patient has consumed can be analysed and preventative advice given. Subsequent diet analysis can be carried out by the patient taking a diet sheet home and filling it out over a four-day period (to include a weekend).

☞ The time between the diet sheet being completed and the next oral heath education appointment should be short so that the patient stays motivated and advice stays relevant.

Diet Analysis

	THURSDAY		FRIDAY		SATURDAY		SUNDAY	
	Time	Item	Time	Item	Time	Item	Time	Item
BEFORE BREAKFAST								
Breakfast								
MORNING								
Mid-day meal								
AFTERNOON								
Evening meal								
EVENING and NIGHT								

Figure 6.8: Diet sheet.

Analysing a diet sheet

☞ It is important to highlight any foods and drinks that contain NMES and noting the frequency with which they are consumed. With each consumption, the plaque pH will fall and an acid attack will occur. The more acid attacks during the day the more demineralisation takes place and the greater the risk of dental caries.

Advice to patient or parents/guardians of patients

Keep sugary foods and drinks to mealtimes only, and try to stick to healthy snacks in-between meals.

☞ It is important to remember that healthy snacks should be healthy for the whole body and not just for teeth, so be aware of fat and salt content too. Enough time must be given between sugary foods and drinks to allow saliva to neutralise the acid and allow remineralisation to occur. For adults, chewing sugar-free gum could be recommended to increase saliva flow.

Advice can be given on hidden sugars, which are sugars added to foods and drinks that may not be immediately obvious, especially in savoury foods. Inform the patient to always read the label and note the ingredients, and any word ending in OSE will denote sugar. The ingredients are listed in amount order. There are products on the market that are known as sugar substitutes and do not cause dental caries. Sugar substitutes include Xylitol, Sorbitol and Mannitol, however, taken in large quantities they can have a laxative effect, especially in children.

Fluoride (DN15.2)

History

The benefits of fluoride have been recorded for some years due to extensive research that began in 1901 with an American dentist called Dr F. McKay. He noticed that the teeth of many of his patients who lived in Colorado Springs had a particular appearance that he called mottled enamel, which showed up as white, yellow, or brown flecks scattered over the surface. However it was not until the 1930s that excessive fluoride in the drinking water, more than 2.0 parts per million fluoride (ppm F) or 2mg F/litre) was shown to be responsible. The patients with mottled enamel also had a low caries experience. This mottling was then called dental fluorosis.

In 1942, Dean and co-workers carried out a study on children aged 12–14 living in 20 towns. This study looked at the relationship between caries experience and the fluoride content of the water supply. The study concluded that 1ppm fluoride in the drinking water resulted in a low caries experience and no dental fluorosis. It also showed that these children had 50% less caries than those with no fluoride in the water. Because of this study the recommended optimum level of fluoride in the water supply is 1ppm in temperate climates and 0.7ppm in tropical climates.

How fluoride can prevent dental caries

Fluoride can be absorbed by the enamel and dentine, making it more resistant to acid attack. Enamel that is more porous, i.e. enamel that has been demineralised, can take up more fluoride than sound enamel. Therefore, it can be beneficial to place fluoride on white or brown spot lesions to help prevent further demineralisation. Enamel from newly erupted teeth takes up more fluoride than mature enamel, and uptake by enamel of calcium and phosphate ions from saliva is improved in the presence of the fluoride ion. Fluoride has also been shown to be toxic to the bacteria *mutans streptococci* which is found in plaque.

Fluoride application

Fluoride can occur naturally in the water supply or be added artificially. Fluoride application can be divided into systemic (taken into the body orally) and topical (applied directly to the tooth).

Systemic

❍ Water – only 10 per cent of the population receives fluoridated water. It can be added at a concentration of 1ppm.

❍ Tablets/drops – if fluoride in water is below 0.3 ppm F then fluoride can be applied as follows:

6-months to 3-years-old – 0.25 mg F daily

3-years to 6-years-old – 0.5mg F daily

6-years and over – 1.0mg F daily

Topical

❍ Toothpaste sodium fluoride/sodium monofluorophosphate ranging from 525 to 1450ppm.

❍ Mouthrinses/gels/varnishes.

Fluorosis

☞ Fluoride supplements should only be prescribed for patients who are at risk from dental caries or where their medical history makes treatment difficult or life threatening. Children under 6 years old should be supervised when brushing their teeth and only a small amount of fluoride toothpaste should be used (small pea size). Fluoride-containing gels and varnishes may be applied in the dental surgery as a preventative measure.

☞ Only the dentist can prescribe fluoride supplements, but a suitably trained DN can provide advice on fluoride and its benefits.

Oral hygiene (DN19.2)

The patient should be advised to brush twice a day with a small-headed, medium-textured toothbrush. Show the patient how to aim the bristles at about a 45° angle to the gingival margin, and if possible, use small circular movements to aid plaque removal and help prevent gingival recession and toothbrush abrasion (see Figure 6.9). Brushing should ideally last for 2–3 minutes, and often, electric toothbrushes can come with timers to help the patient with this.

Brushing alone will not prevent dental caries, and it is important that the patient uses fluoride toothpaste and receives diet advice as well. Advise the patient at risk from caries not to rinse the toothpaste out but just to spit, leaving the toothpaste on the tooth surfaces.

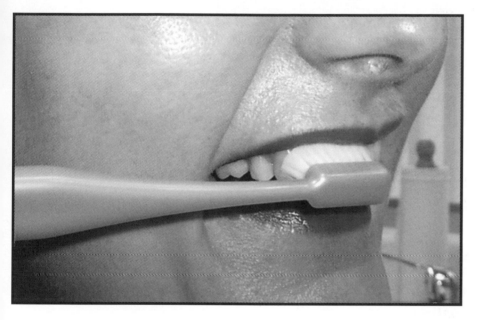

Figure 6.9: Toothbrushing with bristles at 45° angle.

Other oral hygiene measures

Other measures include:

○   single tufted or interspace brush (Figure 6.10(b));

○   interdental or bottle brush (Figure 6.10(c));

○   dental tape/floss (Figure 6.10(d));

When using dental tape or floss it is important the patient is aware that they are cleaning the *sides* of the teeth rather than the space between them. A sliding action is recommended rather than a sawing one.

Regular visits to the dentist

It is advisable for patients to attend the dentist regularly, especially children, so that any dental health problems may be picked up early. This not only includes the early detection of dental caries, but also includes periodontal disease, oral cancer and systemic diseases that may affect the oral cavity.

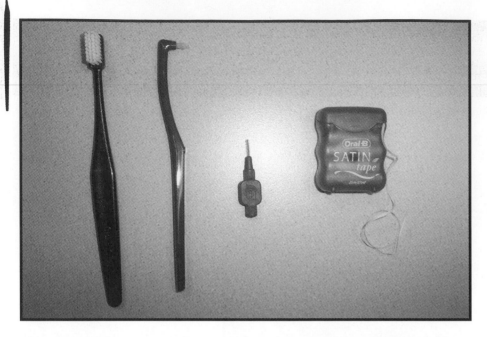

Figure 6.10(a–d): (a) Toothbrush; (b) single tufted or interspace brush; (c) interdental or bottle brush; (d) dental tape.

Fissure sealants (DN15.2)

A fissure sealant may be defined as a material used to seal deep pits and fissures in the permanent molars and premolars. It may also be used to seal deep grooves and developmental pits on the palatal and lingual surfaces of incisors and canines.

☞ Fissure sealants are used as a preventative measure against dental caries, and the teeth most often sealed are the first permanent molars.

Materials used in fissure sealing

The most common material used for fissure sealing is unfilled composite resins. However, glass ionomer and compomers may also be used. Fissure sealants may either be light or chemically cured, and either clear or opaque in appearance. The acid etch technique is used for sealing with unfilled resins.

Indications for fissure sealing

Indications include:

○ Deep pits or fissures

○ High caries experience in patient or siblings

○ Medically compromised patient

○ Learning disability or management problem patient.

Contra indications for fissure sealing

Contra indications include:

○ uncooperative patients

○ poor isolation – it is better not to seal if isolation is poor

○ shallow fissures.

SECTION 3: Periodontal disease linked to DN15

Introduction

This section will cover:

○ The cause of periodontal disease

○ The role of plaque in periodontal disease

○ Diagnosis of periodontal disease

○ Prevention of periodontal disease.

Periodontal disease is a disease of the support structures of the teeth that is primarily caused by plaque. The support structures are:

○ The gingiva

○ The periodontal ligament

○ The alveolar bone

○ The root cementum.

Gingivitis

The first stage of periodontal disease is gingivitis, which can affect up to 95 per cent of the adult population. It is caused by the accumulation of plaque at the gingival margins, which can be lead to an inflammatory response in this tissue. Healthy gingiva is normally pink in colour (with some ethnic variation), stippled, with a tight contoured scalloped edge around the teeth (see Figure 6.11). There is no bleeding on brushing or on using interdental cleaning aids. Gingivitis will cause loss of stippling and contouring due to inflammation of the gingival tissues. The gingiva becomes red and shiny, and bleeding occurs on brushing and using interdental aids (see Figure 6.12).

☞ Gingivitis is a reversible disease and is not normally painful. Due to inflammation of the gingiva a 'false' pocket is created, which will disappear when the oral hygiene improves and the inflammation subsides.

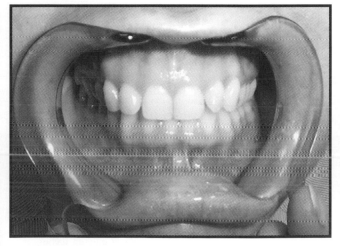

Figure 6.11: Healthy gingiva.

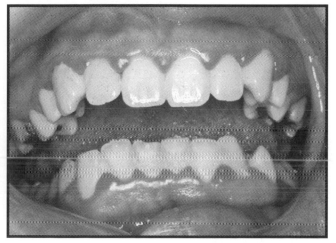

Figure 6.12: Gingivitis.

Periodontitis

☞ Periodontitis is also caused by an accumulation of plaque, but unlike gingivitis it is not reversible and can lead to tooth loss. The plaque bacteria produce toxins that can destroy the periodontal ligament, cementum and alveolar bone (see Figure 6.13). A true pocket is formed that allows more plaque to accumulate deep under the gingiva and against the root surface, making it hard for the patient to clean. Once the support structures are lost the tooth becomes mobile, and if no preventative measures are taken the tooth will eventually be lost. In its later stages, periodontal abscesses can occur and the disease becomes painful. Compared to the 95 per cent of the adult population that suffers from gingivitis, only 8 to 15% of people appear to be at risk from developing periodontitis.

Plaque and periodontal disease (DN19.1 and DN19.2)

Plaque contains about 70 per cent bacteria, and within a short time after brushing it is building up again on the tooth surface, and around the gingival margin. It can build up more in crevices and interdental areas below the contact point – (areas that are more difficult to clean). It also adheres to dentures, crowns, bridges and orthodontic appliances. The longer plaque is allowed to build up the more complex the bacterial content becomes. Aerobic bacteria, (bacteria that like an oxygen-rich environment), are replaced by anaerobic bacteria, (bacteria that do not like oxygen-rich environments).

☞ As the bacteria multiply it attracts more bacteria, and the layer becomes thicker, so that it will be felt by the patient's tongue as a roughness on the teeth, (see Figure 6.14). Plaque can be seen clinically by using disclosing tablets (see Figure 6.15), or by running a blunt probe over the tooth surface.

Bacteria in plaque initially trigger off an inflammatory response in the gingiva, but immune reactions of the patient are also responsible for chronic gingivitis and destructive periodontal disease. The intensity of the reaction will vary from person to person and may fluctuate in the same person both from site to site and with time. The reaction is essentially a defence reaction against plaque micro-organisms and their products.

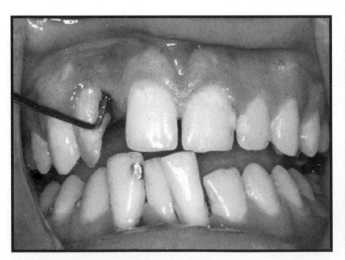

Figure 6.13: Periodontitis.

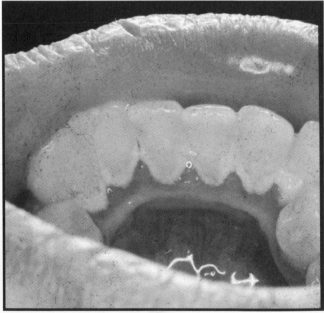

Figure 6.14: Plaque on lingual surface of lower anterior teenth.

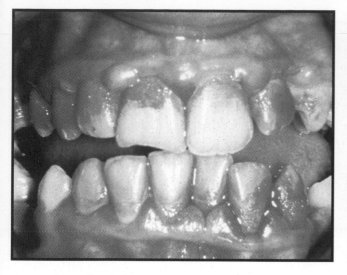

Figure 6.15: Disclosed plaque.

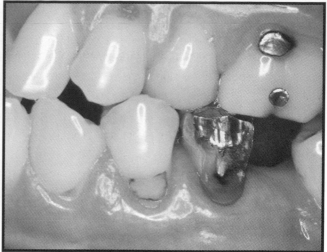

Figure 6.16: Gingival recession with root caries and toothbrush abrasion.

Secondary factors in periodontal disease

Plaque is the primary factor in periodontal disease, but there are also secondary factors that can contribute to it. Secondary factors include host factors, and they may be associated with systemic disease in the patient such as diabetes or Down's syndrome, or by certain drugs. Other factors such as puberty and pregnancy may have an effect on periodontal disease.

Smoking and periodontal disease

Smoking, as well as being associated with cancer and heart disease, has an affect on the periodontal tissues. Patients who smoke tend to have more severe periodontal disease, and do not respond as well to treatment as non-smokers. Smoking can also mask the signs of gingivitis by reducing the amount of bleeding the patient experiences. This is due to the heat from the cigarette constricting the blood vessels near the surface of the gingiva.

Gingival recession

There are two ways in which the gingiva may recede from its normal position around the neck of the tooth. One is due to periodontitis destroying the underlying support structures, and the other is inappropriate brushing. Recession of the gingiva exposes the root surface, which will then be at risk from root caries and toothbrush abrasion (see Figure 6.16). Treatment may include, modification of toothbrushing technique, treatment of the periodontitis and covering the exposed root surface with composite or glass ionomer.

Calculus

Calculus is calcified plaque that adheres to the tooth surface and other objects in the mouth such as dentures, restorations and orthodontic appliances. Although the exact mechanism is not fully understood, saliva deposits calcium and phosphate ions into the plaque, which then becomes calcified. Supra gingival calculus is found above and slightly below the gingival margin and appears as a hard chalky deposit. It builds up mainly on the teeth next to salivary duct openings, which are the lingual surfaces of the lower anterior teeth and the buccal surfaces of the upper molar teeth (see Figure 6.17). Sub gingival calculus forms around all teeth below the gingival margin and is black in colour as blood pigments stain it.

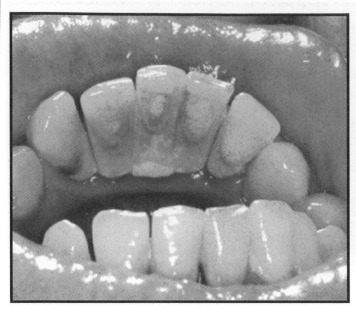

Figure 6.17: Calculus on lingual surface of lower anterior teeth.

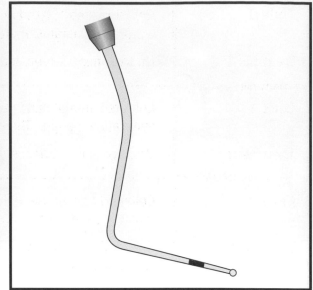

Figure 6.18: A BPE probe.

Diagnosis of periodontal disease

There are many ways of diagnosing periodontal disease, including patient history, direct observation, indices and radiography.

Patient history

The patient may attend the dental surgery because they are concerned by the condition of their teeth and gums. They may have noticed that their gums bleed on brushing, they have halitosis or their teeth are becoming loose. Careful examination and the taking of indices will show how severe their periodontal disease may be and how best to treat it.

Indices (DN15.1)

☞ One index that is used routinely for the screening of periodontal disease is the Basic Periodontal Examination (BPE). This index will give an overall view of the severity of the patient's periodontal disease and the appropriate treatment required. An important aspect of periodontal disease is that is does not always effect the entire mouth in the same way, so some areas may need extensive treatment or surgery and other areas may just need OHE. Other indices tend to be more specific and look at bleeding, plaque accumulation, and mobility. The BPE will now be covered in more detail.

BPE

The BPE probe has a tiny ball at the tip that is 0.5mm in diameter. Along the length of the probe is a black band, which extends from 3.5mm to 5.5.mm (see Figure 6.18). The mouth is then divided up into upper and lower sextants, which define molars and premolars, canines and incisors. The probe is then 'walked' around each tooth and a measurement taken, with only the highest levels recorded for each sextant. Each recorded measurement represents a code and each code represents the treatment required. The codes are given below.

Code 0	Coloured area of band remains completely visible. No calculus or defective restoration margins. There is no bleeding on probing
Treatment	No treatment. Screen again in one year.
Code 1	Coloured area of band remains completely visible. No calculus or defective restoration margins. There is bleeding after gentle probing
Treatment	Oral hygiene instruction. Screen again in one year.
Code 2	Coloured area of the probe remains completely visible. Supra or sub gingival calculus is detected, or there is a defective margin of a restoration.
Treatment	Oral hygiene instruction and removal of calculus and defective restoration margin. Screen again in one year.
Code 3	Coloured area of the probe remains partly visible.
Treatment	As with Code 2, but also it is recommended that plaque and bleeding indices are taken at the beginning and end of treatment. Probing depths should also be taken at the end of treatment in any sextant with a measurement of 3. Screen again in between 6 months to 1 year.
Code 4 or *	Coloured area of probe completely disappears, which indicates a probing depth of over 5.5mm. Once a measurement of 4 is recorded the examiner moves on to the next sextant. A * means there is also furcation involvement (bone loss has reached the lower part of the roots in molars). There may also be recession and probing depths of 7mm or more.
Treatment	A full 6-point pocket chart for that sextant is required. Treatment will also include extensive oral hygiene instruction, deep scaling, removal of any overhangs and defective restoration margins. Periodontal surgery may be required.

Radiographs (DN15.1)

Bitewings, periapical and panoramic radiographs can be used to diagnose bone loss due to periodontitis. Radiographs are a useful teaching tool for the patient, as they can actually see where the bone loss has occurred (see Figure 6.19).

Treatment of periodontal disease

Treatment of periodontal disease may range from simple oral hygiene instruction and supra-gingival scaling on the lower anterior teeth, to extensive periodontal surgery. However, as the primary cause of periodontal disease is plaque it is vital that for any treatment to be successful the patient's oral hygiene must be excellent. Periodontal surgery will not be covered in this chapter.

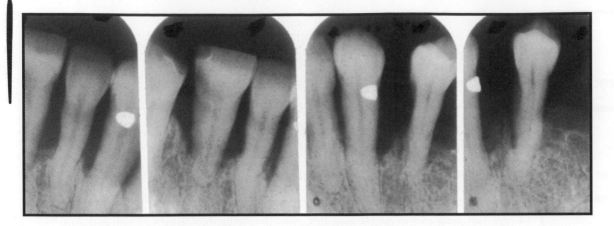

Figure 6.19: Bone loss on periapical radiographs.

Scaling and polishing (DN15.1 and DN15.2)

To remove calculus effectively it is necessary to use professionally designed scaling instruments, and then complete treatment with a polish to make the enamel surface smooth to delay plaque accumulation. Supra-gingival scaling involves removing calculus above, and a little way beneath, the gingival margin. Generally, this treatment should not be too uncomfortable for the patient. Sub-gingival scaling involves removing calculus and plaque below the gingival margins and on the root surface. This treatment can occasionally be uncomfortable and the patient may require a local anaesthetic.

☞ There can be a lot of haemorrhaging during scaling due to gingival inflammation. The DN has an important role to play during treatment by carrying out effective aspiration in order to maintain a clear field of vision and make it more pleasant for the patient.

Scaling instruments (DN15.1 and DN15.2)

Scaling instruments may be divided into hand instruments and sonic/ultrasonic scalers.

Hand scalers

Hand scalers may be divided further into those used supra-gingivally and those used sub-gingivally. There are many scalers available and it is often operator preference that dictates which one is to be used for treatment. Supra-gingival scalers generally have two cutting edges, whist sub-gingival scalers have one, so that they do not damage the pocket lining (see Figure 6.20).

Some supra-gingival and sub-gingival scalers are as follows:

- ❍ Jacquettes – supra-gingival scaling (Figure 20(b))
- ❍ Sickle scalers – supra-gingival scaling (Figure 20(c))
- ❍ Curettes – supra- and sub-gingival scaling (Figure 20(a))
- ❍ Periodontal hoes – sub-gingival scaling (Figure 20(d))

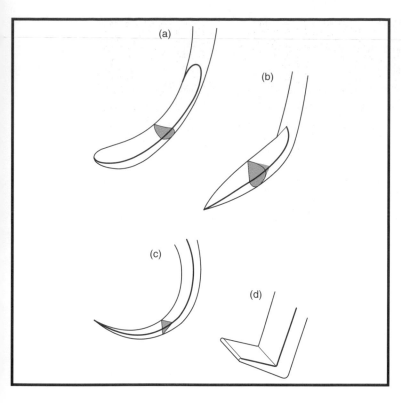

Figure 6.20: Scaling instruments.

Ultrasonic/sonic scalers

Ultrasonic scalers work by the tip oscillating back and forth at a frequency of 25–40 thousand times a second. This movement will result in the mechanical removal of calculus. The tip will get very hot during movement. Therefore, cooling water is passed through the instrument and over the tip, where it meets ultrasonic movement. This ultrasonic movement makes the bubbles in the water oscillate violently, making them implode. This activity results in forces that are capable of shattering calculus.

Sonic scalers work at lower frequencies and are attached to the dental unit's air pressure system (see Figure 6.21). Calculus is removed by vibration of the tip and water is used to cool the tooth surface.

Ultrasonic and sonic tips come in a variety of shapes similar to hand instruments.

Dental hygienists are specially trained to use scaling instruments and the dentist will often refer patients to them.

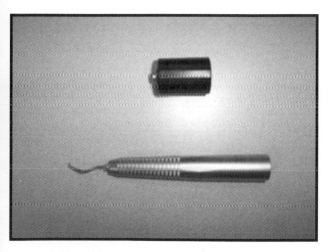

Figure 6.21 Sonic scaler,

Prevention of periodontal diseases

☞ Gingivitis is a reversible disease and health can be restored by the effective, daily removal of plaque. By advising the patient on how to brush effectively and use interdental cleaning aids, the inflammation will subside and bleeding will stop within a short time. However, periodontitis is not reversible, and the aim of preventative treatment is to stabilise the disease and prevent it from progressing. For some patients, they may need extra help by using chemical plaque control such as Chlorhexidene Gluconate 0.2% (Corsodyl) which comes in a mouthwash or gel form. The DN would have to check with the dentist, hygienist or therapist before recommending Chlorhexidene as it does have some side effects, such as staining.

Oral hygiene instruction to the patient would include:

○ Brush twice a day using a small-headed, medium-textured toothbrush.

○ Brush for about three minutes using small circular movements with the bristles aimed at about 45° angle towards the gum margin.

○ Clean the sides between the teeth once a day either using dental floss/tape or an interdental brush.

○ Use disclosing tablets to aid effective cleaning by staining the plaque either blue or red.

○ Remember that bleeding gums are normally a sign of gingivitis, so do not stop brushing or using interdental cleaning aids if you notice any bleeding.

○ Remember that using a mouthwash is no substitute for effective mechanical cleaning.

○ Always consult your dentist or hygienist if symptoms persist.

SECTION 4: The role of the DN in the treatment and prevention of dental caries and periodontal disease

Introduction

This section is linked to DN15.1 and DN15.2 of the NVQ Level 3 in Oral Health Care.

☞ During the preparation of the clinical environment, chairside support nursing and the giving of oral health education, the DN must:

○ be aware of all health and safety issues

○ carry out effective cross infection procedures

○ provide accurate and relevant oral health care advice.

Preparation of clinical area

All surfaces should be disinfected with a solution such as hypochlorite 1.0% (not to be used on metal surfaces). Zone your clinical area into dirty and clean areas and remove any unnecessary items from work surfaces. During this procedure the DN must be wearing protective equipment such as gloves, glasses and mask.

Instruments and materials

The type of instruments and materials being used will, of course, depend on the treatment being carried out. It is the responsibility of the DN to lay out the correct instruments and materials. Two clinical procedures will be highlighted in the scenarios below:

○ Prevention of dental caries

○ Removal of calculus, a polish and oral hygiene instruction.

Scenario 1

Fissure sealants in all first permanant molars

An example for the prevention of dental caries is as follows.

The patient is 6 years old, and they have had a high caries rate in their deciduous teeth. Their older sibling, who is 8 years old, has had restorations in both lower permanent first molars. There is no sign of caries as yet, so fissure sealants are recommended as a preventative measure. A dentist, therapist or hygienist may carry out this procedure.

Lay out instruments:

○ Mirror, straight probe, tweezers.

○ Flat plastic.

Lay out handpieces and polishing cups/brushes:

○ Contra angled (slow) handpiece.

○ Polishing cup or brush.

Lay out rubber dam equipment:

Fissure sealing is best carried out under rubber dam for health and safety and good isolation.

○ Rubber dam sheet

○ Rubber dam hole punch

○ Rubber dam clamp forceps

○ Rubber dam clamps for lower molars (the tooth behind the one being treated is often clamped)

○ Rubber dam frame

○ Dental floss for holding the clamp

Lay out local anaesthetic equipment:

LA may have to be given to make the clamp more comfortable.

○ Check with the dentist regarding the patient's medical history first to see if there is any contra indication to adrenaline or octapressin

○ Topical anaesthetic

○ Local anaesthetic cartridge

○ Short local anaesthetic needle and self-aspirating syringe

Lay out materials for etching the tooth:

○ Etchant liquid.

○ Dappens pot.

○ Applicator brush.

○ Cotton wool rolls/pledgets.

Materials for sealing the tooth:

○ Unfilled composite resin.

○ Plastic applicator.

○ Light curing machine (cover tip in clear plastic protective sheet for infection control).

○ Protective shield.

Lay out other items including:

○ Articulating paper to check occlusion for high spots.

○ Fluoride varnish to place over any etched area not sealed.

○ Non-fluoride prophy paste or pumice and water mix.

○ Aspirating tips.

○ Air/water tips.

○ Gauze squares.

○ Protective glasses for the patient, dentist and DN.

○ Protective bib for the patient.

○ Gloves and masks for the dentist and DN.

☞ Chairside support

Prior to procedure:

○ All instruments should really be covered with a clean paper towel before use so they are out of sight of the patient and protected from dust particles or other contamination.

○ Fit the handpiece into its connector.

○ Place aspirators into tubing and safely load the syringe.

○ Welcome the patient (and parent/guardian if necessary) into the surgery.

○ Ask patient to sit in the chair and protect them with a bib and glasses.

○ Make sure you and the operator are wearing all protective equipment before the procedure begins.

Giving LA:

○ Place some topical anaesthetic onto a cotton wool roll or pledget and pass to the dentist.

○ Pass the loaded syringe with the needle cap in place to the dentist. Never pass it with the needle ungarded and never pass it over the patient's face or in their line of vision.

○ Monitor patient throughout the giving of the LA and give support if the patient is nervous by holding their hand for example.

○ Ensure the needle is re-sheathed by the dentist. The nurse must never re-sheathe a needle, and unsheathed needles must never be left on the tray or work surfaces.

Placement of rubber dam:

○ Pass the dentist a length of floss so they can clean around the contact points of the tooth to be clamped.

○ Place a piece of floss around the clamp, place it in the forceps and pass to the dentist.

○ Punch the appropriate holes into the rubber dam sheet and pass to the dentist.

○ Assist with placing the rubber dam sheet over the clamp, flossing it down beneath the contact points and blowing air to aid inversion of the sheet.

○ Assist with placing the frame and check the patient can breathe freely and is comfortable. A small piece of sheet may need to be cut around the patient's nose to make breathing more comfortable.

○ Provide the patient with a flexible saliva ejector that they can use under the rubber dam.

Etching and sealing the tooth

○ Pass the dentist pumice or prophy in a dappens pot.

○ After the tooth has been polished aspirate whist the operator washes the tooth.

○ Place the etchant in a dappens pot and pass to the dentist with a brush (never pass over the patient's face).

○ Aspirate whilst the dentist is washing away etchant.

○ Dry tooth thoroughly.

○ Place sealant in dappens pot and pass to dentist with applicator.

○ Hold protective shield whilst the dentist light cures sealant.

○ Monitor patient throughout procedure.

Completion of procedure:

○ Assist in removing the rubber dam.

○ Wipe patient's mouth clean of saliva and any debris.

○ Pass the dentist articulating paper.

○ Place fluoride varnish on pad and pass with flat plastic.

○ Make sure patient is happy to leave surgery and arrange another appointment if necessary.

Cleaning of clinical environment after procedure:

○ Dispose of all sharps in sharps bin.

○ Dispose of all clinical waste in yellow clinical waste bag.

○ Clean instruments of saliva, blood and debris in ultrasonic bath and/or scrub under water with long-handled brush and wearing thick gloves, a mask and glasses.

○ Oil handpiece.

○ Remove excess water from instruments and place evenly on a perforated tray.

○ Place tray into autoclave for sterilisation.

☞ If rubber dam is not being used it is essential that good isolation of the tooth and protection of the patient are carried out. The DN plays a vital role in making sure that:

○ There is good isolation and protection of soft tissues from acid etch.

○ There is excellent aspiration to prevent inhalation or swallowing of acid etch.

○ The face and eyes are protected from acid etch.

○ There is protection of clothes from acid etch.

○ Eye protection for patient, DN and operator from light.

Scenario 2

The removal of calculus, a polish and oral health instruction

The patient has complained of bleeding on brushing, and they have noticed some calculus build-up around their lower front teeth, which they can feel with their tongue. A simple supra-gingival scale and polish followed by oral hygiene instruction is recommended.

Lay out instruments:

○ Mirror, probe, (straight, periodontal measuring and BPE), tweezers.

○ Selection of handscalers including, sickle scalers, curettes, jacquette.

Lay out handpiece and ultrasonic/sonic scalers and tips:

○ Contra angled (slow) handpiece.

○ Prophy cup/brush.

Lay out other items including:

○ Prophy paste.

○ Dappens pot.

○ Toothbrush.

○ Dental tape/floss.

○ Selection of interdental cleaners.

○ Hand mirror.

○ Disclosing tablets.

○ Aspirating tips.

○ Air/water tips.

○ Cotton wool rolls and pledgets.

○ Gauze squares.

○ Protective glasses for the patient, dentist and DN.

○ Protective bib for the patient.

○ Gloves and masks for the dentist and DN.

☞ Chairside support

Prior to procedure:

○ All instruments should really be covered with a clean paper towel before use so they are out of sight of the patient and protected from dust particles or other contamination.

○ Fit the handpiece and ultrasonic/sonic scaling tips into their connectors.

○ Place aspirators into tubing.

○ Welcome the patient into the chair and protect them with a bib and glasses.

○ Make sure you and the dentist are wearing all protective equipment before the procedure begins.

Disclosing the patient:

○ The operator may wish to disclose the patient first to check oral hygiene.

○ Give patient disclosing tablet to chew.

○ Provide the patient with a rinse (only one short rinse).

○ Hold hand mirror so the operator can show the patient the area covered in plaque.

Scaling:

○ Pass the operator hand scaling instruments.

○ Aspirate blood, calculus and debris from patient's mouth.

○ Aspirate water and calculus when ultrasonic/sonic scaler is being used.

○ Monitor patient at all times.

Completion of procedure:

○ Wipe patient's mouth clean of saliva and any debris.

○ Allow patient to rinse.

○ If requested by operator and you are suitably trained then you can give the patient oral hygiene instruction.

○ Show them an effective brushing and interdental cleaning technique. First show on a model then get the patient to demonstrate in their own mouth.

○ Remember each patient has individual oral health needs and oral health instruction should reflect that fact.

○ If the patient struggles with floss then try interdental brushes.

○ If the patient finds it hard to move the brush in small circular movements then maybe recommend a power toothbrush.

○ Make sure patient is happy to leave surgery and arrange another appointment if necessary.

Cleaning of clinical environment after procedure:

○ Dispose of all sharps in sharps bin.

○ Dispose of all clinical waste in yellow clinical waste bag.

○ Clean instruments of saliva, blood and debris in ultrasonic bath and/or scrub under water with long-handled brush and wearing thick gloves, a mask and glasses.

○ Oil handpieces.

○ Remove excess water from instruments and place evenly on a perforated tray.

○ Place tray into autoclave for sterilisation.

SECTION 5: The DN's role in prevention of dental caries and periodontal disease

This section is linked to DN19.1, DN19.2, DN19.3, DN19.4 of the NVQ Level 3 in Oral Health Care.

☞ A suitably trained DN can provide the patient with information on preventing caries and periodontal disease. A separate session can be arranged for the patient to attend for oral health education (OHE) or it can be carried out on the day of treatment.

Environment

○ A surgery, or a separate room designated for OHE can be used.

○ Have educational resources available such as models, toothbrushes, pictures, leaflets and diet sheets.

○ Make sure that there is adequate lighting, space and comfortable seating and that you will not be disturbed during the session.

OHE session

○ Make out a lesson plan before the session, stating aims and objectives and areas that you will cover.

○ Do not make the session too long, or try to get too much information across in one go.

○ Assess the patient's previous knowledge by asking relevant questions.

○ Always address the patient's individual needs, taking into account such factors as age, socio-economic status (e.g. would they be able to afford expensive electric toothbrushes), medical history (e.g. do they have special needs), dental status (e.g. do they wear dentures or have a bridge).

○ Assess the patient's learning by asking them to demonstrate techniques you have shown them.

○ You can evaluate a session by the use of a questionnaire or asking questions.

Follow-up sessions

○ Reassess what the patient has learnt from the last session by asking questions.

○ Reinforce the preventative message.

○ Check with the dentist for any new carious lesions or check periodontal indices to monitor patient's clinical progress.

Dental caries and periodontal disease are the world's most common diseases, and both are preventable. A trained DN, in giving appropriate and realistic preventative advice, will help patients to avoid pain, tooth loss and invasive dental treatment.

References

[1] Committee on Medical Aspects (of food policy) (COMA).

[2] Kidd, E.A.M. and Joyston-Bechal, S, *Essentials of Dental Caries.* (1997); 2nd Edition; Oxford.

[3] Manson J.E, *An outline of periodontics*. (1983) 1st Edition; Wright.

[4] Waite I.M. and Strahan J.D, *A colour atlas of periodontology*. (1990); 2nd Edition; Wolfe.

[5] Williams D.M, Hughes F.J., Odell E.W. and Farthing P.M, *Pathology of periodontal diseases*. (1992); 1st Edition; Oxford Medical Publications.

[6] Brand and Isselhard, *Anatomy of oralfacial structures*. (1994); 5th Edition; Mosby.

[7] Levison H., *Textbook for dental nurses*. (1997); 8th Edition; Blackwell Science.

[8] Millward M.R. and Chapple I.L.C., Classification of periodontal diseases: Where were we? Where are we now? Where are we going? *Dental Update*; January/February 2003; 37–44.

[9] Ower, Philip *The role of Self-Administration Plaque Control in the Management of Periodontal Diseases* Paper 1 – A Review of Evidence March 2003, 60–66.

7 CONSERVATION

Introduction

This chapter is linked to DN15.1, 15.1.3, 21.1.23 and 20.2 of the NVQ Level 3 in Oral Health Care.

SECTION 1:   Caries linked to DN15.1

Dental caries is a disease that affects the calcified parts of the teeth, namely enamel, dentine and cementum (see Figure 7.1).

Enamel

○ Makes up the surface of the coronal part of the tooth.

○ The hardest tissue found in the body.

○ Made up of approximately 97 per cent by weight of mineral compound. This compound is known as hydroxyapatite. It contains phosphorus and a high content of calcium. It has a microscopic 'rod' or 'prism' formation held together with interprismatic substances. As it contains no nerve tissue it is insensitive.

Dentine

○ A calcified material, which makes up most of the crown and root. Like enamel, it is made up of the compound hydroxyapatite and is approximately 70 per cent of mineral compound.

○ It is not as hard as enamel and there are fine tubules containing fibrils, which transmit sensations and are therefore able to transmit pain.

Cementum

○ A structure much like bone.

○ A thin layer covers the dentine on the surface of the root.

○ A connective tissue in which the periodontal ligaments are attached.

○ The percentage of mineral compound is not known exactly.

Process

The process of caries starts when the bacteria *streptococci mutans* and *lactobacillus* (which are present in dental plaque) come into contact with fermentable carbohydrates in food. Examples of these carbohydrates include: glucose, sucrose, fructose, lactose and cooked starches. After a period of time, of around 1–3 minutes, these bacteria produce acid. This acid reacts firstly with the enamel and then the dentine. The rate at which the bacteria produce the acid can depend on the type of carbohydrate, glucose and sucrose having the most rapid rate.

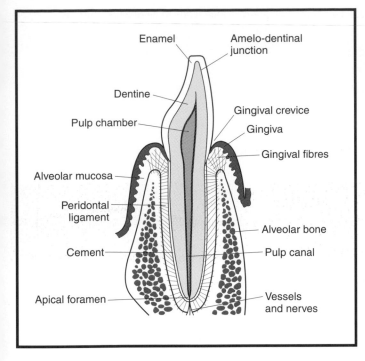

Figure 7.1: The anatomy of the tooth.

This initial stage is of caries is known as demineralisation and the first sign is a 'white spot'. A cavity has not yet formed at this stage and the tooth still has a hard surface. If demineralisation is left to continue, not reversed by the action of saliva or fluoride applications, and there is frequent sugar consumption, the acid further dissolves the calcified tissues of the enamel and a 'lesion' forms. The disease then progresses through the dentine and may reach the pulp. This leads to pulp inflammation (pulpitis), infection and possible pulp death (necrosis).

There are other factors that affect the progression of dental caries. For example, when *streptococcus mutans* and *lactobacillus* bacteria in dental plaque come into contact with fermentable carbohydrates they produce acid. Acidity is expressed in terms of the concentration of hydrogen ions and is denoted using 'pH'. The pH of 7 is neutral, higher than 7 is alkaline and less than 7 is acidic. The usual pH level in the mouth is around 7. The plaque changes from its normal level of 7 and drops to somewhere between 4 and 5 after only a couple of minutes. Decalcification of tooth tissue begins when the pH drops below 5.5. This can be illustrated using a 'Stephan Curve' (see Figure 7.2).

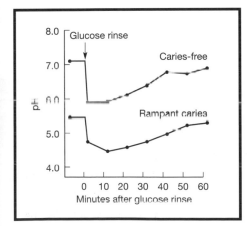

Figure 7.2: Changes in pH in plaque following a glucose rinse, the Stephan Curve.

The areas of tooth tissue where dental caries most frequently occurs are those where the plaque tends to be retained, such as stagnation areas. Examples of these areas are:

○ Fissures on molars and premolars

○ Pits, for example, buccal of 1st molars and anteriors palatally

○ Interdentally at the contact area

○ Cervical surfaces

○ Root surfaces – related to gingival recession

○ Around defective restorations including overhangs.

Diagnosis

The diagnosis of dental caries can be made using routine clinical methods such as direct vision, as tooth tissue appears discoloured.

Deficiencies on the tooth surface can be detected using a straight probe. Ensuring that the condition would not be made worse the probe may stick into an affected site. Also, any demineralisation or carious lesions that are not visible by direct vision may be evident with transmitted light or on radiographs such as intra-oral bitewings.

Treatment

Caries is usually treated by surgical removal as in cavity preparation. Examples of preventative measures that reduce the caries rate considerably include:

○ Patient education

○ Regular visits to the dentist and dental hygienist

○ Fluoride and fissure-sealant treatments.

Caries rate

Treatment depends on the caries rate. The calcium and phosphate ions contained in saliva have an effect on the progress of caries. The saliva neutralises the acid attack and causes the tooth tissue to repair or remineralise to a certain extent. This is providing that the frequencies of the other factors that cause caries are reduced, (such as sugar intake). This would be regarded as **arrested** caries. The caries process often alternates between demineralising and remineralising and continues over a period of months, sometimes before actual lesions appear.

The rapid rate is known as **rampant** caries and, apart from being often found in very young children with primary dentition who have been given bottles containing sugary drinks, it is also found in teenagers and those whose diet includes frequent snacking on foods containing fermentable carbohydrates.

The type of caries that affects the root surface is known as **root caries** and tends to develop at a faster rate than that forming on the coronal part of the tooth structure. This is because the root is not covered by the hard tissue of enamel, but is comprised of the softer dentine. Therefore, the demineralisation process is more rapid. This 'root caries' is often associated with adults who have gingival recession.

The caries rate is greatly influenced by the contents of saliva and its rate of flow. A reduction in the rate of salivary flow is known as **xerostomia**. Saliva contains minerals and antibacterial agents that, together, have an effect on bacteria levels and aid the remineralisation process.

There are circumstances that affect saliva contents and the rate of flow. Xerostomia is evident during sleep and is related to the ageing process. It is also related to the side effects of certain drug treatments including radiotherapy.

QUESTIONS

Question 1

a. What are the four factors that cause dental caries?

b. Name the bacteria that cause dental caries.

c. At what level of pH does the decalcification of teeth begin?

d. Name six stagnation areas.

e. Name three types of caries, relating to its progress.

f. Name the condition that is associated with a 'dry mouth'.

SECTION 2:   Restoration of cavities Linked to DN15.1.3

The destruction of tooth tissue due to dental caries is often the reason for the restoration of a cavity. The cavity is filled with the most appropriate restorative material for that particular circumstance. This restores the tooth to its original function. The treatment might also be necessary following loss of tooth tissue as a result of tooth wear and trauma.

Dental caries

The usual treatment of a carious lesion is the surgical removal of the caries and the lost tooth tissue is replaced by a filling material.

Tooth wear

The three main types of tooth wear are erosion, abrasion and attrition.

Erosion of the tooth surface can be caused by:

○ Acids found in foods such as fruit and carbonated drinks.

○ Food being constantly regurgitated, as in the case of certain medical conditions.

○ Acid found in some general working environments. This cause can be avoided by wearing the correct personal protective equipment.

Abrasion can occur on the tooth surface following:

- Long-term ingestion of abrasive foodstuffs.
- Use of an excessively hard toothbrush or very abrasive toothpaste.

Attrition is the loss of the tooth surface due to tooth-to-tooth contact such as grinding (bruxism).

Trauma

The loss of tooth tissue due to trauma is not a slow process but sudden. Injuries can occur:

- In a fall, during a sporting activity.
- As a result of violence.
- During a sporting activity.

☞ Surgery procedure

The branch of dentistry dealing with the diagnosis, prevention and treatment of diseases of the enamel and dentine is known as 'Operative Dentistry'. As with all specialities in dentistry it requires that the dental nurse (DN) has a detailed knowledge of the various procedures in order to be an efficient chairside assistant. Some of the many reasons for having this efficient support includes the saving of surgery time during a procedure, stress for the dentist is reduced and the job satisfaction of the DN is increased.

Preparation

It is important to wash hands thoroughly and prepare all items necessary for the procedure. All working areas should be cleared of any unnecessary items and the work surfaces (and any area that may be contaminated during the treatment) should be wiped down with an appropriate disinfection solution.

Patient records

The next stage is to select the appropriate patient records, including radiographs, and lay out the instruments and materials necessary. Dentists have their own preference with regard to items and it is important to familiarise yourself with them.

Instrument placement

To maintain an efficient working environment, instruments should be set up in the order of use. This logical order makes the transfer of instruments during the procedure easier. With the knowledge of the procedure and a tray set up in a logical order, the DN needs to anticipate every stage. This enables the procedure to progress efficiently and effectively and the patient will be aware of the quality of treatment that they are receiving. It may also reduce any patient anxiety.

Surgery furniture

Once the instruments and materials are laid out in an area that is easily accessible to the team, it is important to place the operator chair and DN chair in the appropriate position and height for ease of work.

Patient seating

The patient is greeted in the waiting area by the DN and escorted to the surgery where they are asked to sit in the dental chair safely and comfortably. The DN may need to adjust the chair and headrest.

The patient's chair is in the upright position for the initial welcoming so that the dentist and patient can communicate face to face. The dentist consults with the patient regarding changes in medical history and any reports from the previous visit. The required treatment to be undertaken is discussed and, with mutual agreement, the treatment commences.

The DN informs the patient that the chair is to be placed in the supine position and they are supplied with a protective 'bib' for clothing. Protective eyewear is also provided as the eyes are more vulnerable while the patient is supine and prevents any 'foreign bodies' coming into contact with them during the procedure.

The dentist and DN wash their hands and put on their eyewear, mask and gloves. The dental team should wear gloves when coming into contact with potential contaminants and wear protective eyewear and masks when contaminated aerosols are present.

Prior to putting on the personal protective equipment it is important to wash hands for at least one minute using an antiseptic handwashing agent. This simple routine reduces the risk of cross infection.

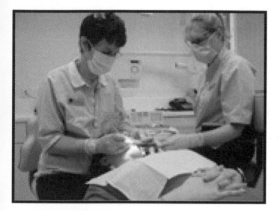

Figure 7.3: Positioning of the dentist and dental nurse for the start of procedure.

👉 Instrumentation

The following items may be needed for an amalgam filling:

- Dental mouth mirror (front surface) for indirect vision, light reflection, soft tissue retraction.

- Straight probe for the careful detection of caries.

- College tweezers for the transference of small items e.g. cotton wool pledgets.

- Excavators (small/large) with discoid (round) or cleoid (pear shaped) blades for removal of soft caries, insertion of linings and carving amalgam.

- Gingival margin trimmers (distal/mesial) and enamel chisels for removal of unsupported enamel.

- Flat plastic for insertion and shaping of materials.

- Amalgam condenser for condensing material within the cavity.

- Amalgam carvers for the removal of excess material and shaping amalgam.

- Amalgam burnishers (ball ended) for smoothing amalgam after carving.

- Cavity lining applicator for the insertion of some cavity linings.

- Cement spatula for mixing cements.

- Amalgam carrier for the insertion of amalgam into cavity.

- Items for administration of local anaesthetic.

- Items for the control of the operating field including the application of rubber dam.

- Air/water syringe.

- Aspirator tip.

- Cotton wool rolls.

- Cotton wool pellets.

- 'Dry-guards'.

- 'Dry-tips'.

- Saliva ejectors.

☞ The following rubber dam equipment may be needed

- Rubber dam sheet – 15cm square rubber sheet that grips the teeth and retracts the gingiva.

- Rubber dam hole punch – the size of the hole should depend on the size of the tooth. A perfectly round hole without tags should avoid tearing during application.

- Rubber dam clamp forceps – used to apply, adjust and remove rubber dam clamps.

- Rubber dam clamps – available in many shapes and sizes to fit all teeth.

- Rubber dam frame – various types are available. It holds the edges and corners of the sheet away from the mouth to aid visibility.

- Dental floss – attached to the clamp for safety purposes in the event that the bow of the clamp may snap; helps in the placement of the sheet around teeth in the contact point area.

- Rubber dam lubricant – water soluble substance that can be placed on the inside surface of the rubber sheet to enable the sheet to slip easily over the teeth.

- Gauze napkins – place between the rubber sheet and patient's skin for comfort.

- Scissors – to cut a wedge of rubber to anchor the sheet in position; to cut the interdental part of the rubber sheet prior to its removal.

- Handpieces – air rotor (used in conjunction with friction grip burs at high speed (approximately 100,000 RPM) for the removal of enamel and dentine); conventional motor (used in conjunction with latch grip burs at a slow speed (approximately 10,000 RPM with possible reduction to as slow as 1000 RPM with a special reduction handpiece) for the removal of hard caries. Also used with a friction grip head and burs for cavity modifications and the finishing of restorative materials).

- Intra coronal burs – friction grip diamond burs; friction grip tungsten carbide burs; latch-grip bur for the removal of caries.

- Matrices – include matrix retainers; metal bands; transparent bands; soft metal matrices for gingival cervical cavities; used to re-contour the tooth.

- Wooden wedges – used in conjunction with matrix bands.

○ Lining materials – various types mentioned later in this section.

○ Amalgam capsules – as above.

○ Articulating paper – coloured marking paper used to check that the patient is closing their teeth together in the correct occlusion. High spots of a restoration are highlighted as coloured marks on the tooth when the patient bites on the paper.

Control of the operating field

The mouth generally has many inaccessible places and there is always the problem of moisture. Most materials used in dentistry are detrimentally affected by the presence of moisture. These problems can be overcome with an understanding of how to control the operating field.

Visibility can be improved with suitable light sources and magnification. Also, indirect vision and light reflection using the dental mouth mirror along with the retraction of the soft tissues (i.e. lips, cheeks, tongue) can help.

The control of saliva can be achieved using **absorbent materials**, such as **cotton wool rolls**, which are placed often buccally to the upper right or left first molar. It is in this area that Stenson's duct from the parotid salivary gland transports saliva into the mouth.

For the lower arch, cotton wool rolls are placed buccally and lingually. There are numerous tiny salivary ducts from the sublingual salivary gland on the floor of the mouth under the tongue with two larger ducts from the submandibular salivary gland. The larger are called Wharton's ducts.

Dry-guards or **dry-tips** can be used instead of cotton wool rolls in appropriate areas in the region of the Stenson's duct. They are pads made of absorbent materials.

In addition to saliva, water is produced by the air rotor for cooling purposes. This is to prevent the overheating of the tooth tissue, which could lead to pulpal damage or its death. The presence of water collecting in the mouth is uncomfortable to the patient. It also can pose a problem in tooth preparation and during the use of restorative materials.

Other products of tooth preparation such as tooth debris and filling debris, along with blood from the gingiva or pulp, are regarded as contaminants and need to be removed. The control of these contaminants can be achieved using **high or low volume suction** connected to a suitable **aspirator tip**. An **air/water syringe** can be used in conjunction with the aspirator tip to wash and dry the cavity, and to remove the debris. The use of the air/water syringe without use of the aspirator tip can add to the problem of moisture control.

A **saliva ejector** can also be attached to the suction apparatus for the removal of moisture build-up in the floor of the mouth. Some are disposable tubes that can be modified in shape, placed lingually and held in place by the patient. A metal flanged saliva ejector can be placed lingually and, in addition to removing moisture build-up, the flange helps retract the tongue and can act as a mirror to a certain extent, which may aid visibility.

The tongue often seems to have a mind of its own and an extraordinary ability to seek out a revolving bur, aspirator tip or dry cavity. Therefore one of the many duties of the DN is to be constantly aware of its position.

The most effective method for controlling the operating field is with the use of **rubber dam** which isolates the treatment area. The reasons to use a rubber dam include:

○ Prevents inhalation of debris and small items.

○ Prevents swallowing debris and small items.

○ Helps retract soft tissues.

○ Aids in the prevention of moisture contamination of restorative materials.

○ Maintains a dry operating field.

○ Helps improve the comfort of the patient.

There are many ways to apply a rubber dam. Here is one example.

○ A hole or holes are made in a rubber sheet using a rubber dam hole punch by the DN. You must ensure that the holes are clean cut with no tears.

○ A rubber dam clamp with dental floss attached is placed on a tooth using a pair of rubber dam clamp forceps.

○ The hole in the rubber dam sheet that corresponds with the clamped tooth is carefully stretched over the bow of the clamp, and then eased over one side of the clamp and then the other. The clamped tooth is then isolated. The remaining teeth are also eased through each hole.

○ Dental floss is used to ease the rubber interdentally.

○ The edges and corners of the sheet are stretched over a rubber dam frame by the DN.

○ The DN may sometimes put a gauze napkin under the sheet where it is in contact with the patient's skin, for their comfort.

○ The patient should be able to continue to swallow once the rubber dam has been applied, but if they have difficulties then a disposable saliva ejector can be placed under the sheet, in the floor of the mouth, to remove any saliva that collects in that area.

Cavity preparation

Once local anaesthesia has been achieved (if necessary) and the chosen method of saliva control is in place the dentist then gains access to the caries by removing a quantity of enamel and dentine. This is done using an air rotor with a cutting bur. During this stage, the DN keeps the area clear of debris and fluids using the high volume suction and aspirator tip. If a rubber dam is not being used, the aspirating tip is used to retract the soft tissue that may inhibit the view of the dentist. Apart from using the dental mouth mirror for reflecting light, the dentist may also use the mirror for soft tissue retraction.

The DN can use the air/water syringe in conjunction with the aspirator tip to clear the cavity of debris and also to clear the mirror surface.

Once the dentist has opened up the cavity, the DN, if within reach of the instruments, can pass the excavators that are used to remove soft caries. Any harder caries that needs to be removed can be done so using a conventional contra-angled handpiece with a rose-head (round) bur. The aim is to remove soft caries and that which is around the amelo-dentinal junction. This is where the enamel meets the dentine. The dentist determines whether any areas that have arrested caries or staining can remain.

The cavity is then modified using hand instruments (e.g. gingival margin trimmers or chisels) passed by the DN, and burs (e.g. fissure burs). The DN continues to keep the area clear using the air/water syringe and aspirator.

Cavity lining

Once the cavity preparation has been completed a decision is made as to whether the placement of a lining material is beneficial. If the cavity is minimal then the pulp will be protected from chemical, mechanical and thermal irritation by the dentine. In deeper cavities, a lining is needed to protect the pulp. This lining will:

○ promote secondary dentine

○ protect against thermal changes

○ protect against chemical irritants of some restorative materials (e.g. composite resin).

Linings may also be used to strengthen a tooth that is structurally weak and to aid the adhesion of certain restorative materials. Lining materials include:

○ calcium hydroxide

○ glass ionomer cement

○ cavity varnish.

There are numerous lining materials available and it is important for the DN to collect the relevant manufacturer's instructions and the material safety data sheets (MSDS). These would need to be stored and easily retrievable, not only to ensure that the materials are prepared as the manufacturers suggest but also for health and safety reasons.

Calcium hydroxide is a cavity lining material that is used as a protective liner under restorative materials such as amalgam and composite resin; or as a sub-lining for other cavity lining materials. It can be radiopaque, which means that it is visible on a radiograph. This ensures that the lining will not appear as a void and therefore will not be mistaken for dental disease. It also helps to stimulate the formation of secondary dentine, which will protect the pulp and maintain its vitality.

It is presented in tubes as a two-paste system. One tube contains the base and the other contains the catalyst. Mixing involves the DN placing equal amounts of base and catalyst paste on a suitable mixing pad and immediately combining the two pastes using a cement spatula until a homogenous mix is achieved. This is when the white colour of the base and the cream colour of the catalyst become a uniform shade. The **mixing time** should be within **10 seconds**.

Placement of the material requires a specialised hand instrument with a small ball on its end. This instrument is handed to the dentist and the prepared material on the pad is held by the DN within easy reach of the dentist. The small ball on the end of the instrument takes up a small quantity of the material, which is then flowed onto the base of the cavity.

Working and setting time will be faster in the mouth than on the mixing pad because of the increased temperature and moisture. It may take **less than 2¹/₂**. The dentist may need to remove excess material and this can be done using an excavator or probe.

Glass ionomer cements that can be used in deep cavities as a lining have been specially designed for use under amalgam or composite resin and need to be over a sub-lining of calcium hydroxide. They bond to dentine and releases fluoride. It should be designed to be radiopaque for the reason mentioned in the previous section concerning calcium hydroxide. They aid in the protection of the pulp and improves the structure of a weakened tooth.

An example of a glass ionomer is presented in capsulated form and, once mechanically mixed, is used with a dispensing device.

Cavity conditioning involves a cavity or dentine conditioner being applied to the bonding surfaces of the tooth using a cotton wool pellet or suitable applicator. This is left on the surface for either **10** or **20 seconds** depending on the conditioner and then rinsed and dried thoroughly with air/water syringe and aspirator tip.

Capsule preparation immediately before mixing can require the DN to tap the capsule against the work surface to loosen up the powder, push the capsule plunger and place the capsule in a specialised device that activates the capsule. **Mixing** takes place in an amalgamator for a period of 10 seconds. Immediately after mixing, the DN places the capsule in an applicator, adjusts the nozzle direction depending on the position of the tooth to be treated and hands it to the dentist.

Placement of the material is by squeezing the applicator so that the material is dispensed directly into the cavity. Working time is one and a quarter minutes for a fast capsule and 2 minutes for a standard capsule. Setting time is two minutes for the fast set and two minutes 20 seconds for the standard set.

Finishing of the material can be carried out approximately **3** minutes after the start of mixing using suitable burs.

On completion of the lining the DN is then able to dismantle the various devices, dispose of empty capsules and clear away items that will not be needed for the next stage.

Cavity varnishes have been used to help prevent bacteria and microleakage into the dentine tubules affecting the margin of tooth and the filling material. They are resin materials in a solvent liquid.

A very small amount of liquid is placed in a dappens pot immediately before it is needed. If it is left for too long in the air it will evaporate rapidly.

Placement is directly into the cavity with an appropriate applicator and setting time is almost immediate if the layer is thin. Once the chosen lining(s) have been inserted and the cavity is clean and dry the tooth is ready for the permanent restoration. The placement of a matrix may be needed at this stage and if the restoration requires additional retention it may be necessary to place pins.

Pins

Dental materials have improved much over the years with regard to replacing the weakened structure of teeth and providing increased retention for permanent restorations.

Many dentists improve the retention of plastic restorations by cutting slots or grooves, but there may still be occasions for the use of pins. They are used with the appropriate sized bur or twist drill in a slow speed contra-angled handpiece that creates a hole for the pin to be placed. The pin hole is made in the most appropriate place for optimum retention and well away from any possibility of exposing the pulp or periodontal membrane. The DN removes any debris from the hole using air from the air/water syringe. Using the example of the self-shearing technique, the pin, which has a special fitment for the contra-angled handpiece, is placed in the pin hole and the handpiece rotates it so, once the pin has reached the required level, it separates from the latch grip base.

Matrices

○ Used to re-create the original anatomical shape of the missing tooth surface.

○ Produce a good contact point and prevent the excess of restorative material and so reduce the risk of overhangs.

○ Save time at the finishing stage.

○ Metal bands are used in a matrix retainer prior to the insertion of amalgam.

○ Metal bands also available without retainers but are supplied with special applicators and removers.

○ Soft metal matrices can be used for the insertion of chemically cured glass ionomers in a gingival cervical cavity.

○ Transparent bands can be used for the insertion of composite resins, as they do not hinder the light-curing.

○ Transparent crown forms are also available to be used with materials such as composite resin.

Wooden wedges

○ Used in conjunction with matrix bands to hold the bands in place and for the reasons mentioned above.

○ For light-curing materials transparent wedges are needed.

Filling insertion

Amalgam

This material is used in the case of cavities in posterior teeth that have occlusal contact. Occlusal contact is the relationship that the upper arch of teeth has with the lower arch on closing together, biting and chewing. In this case it is important to have a strong durable material able to withstand load-bearing situations. Due to the appearance of amalgam it is not suitable aesthetically for anterior restorations.

Matrix placement may be necessary in the event of a cavity with missing walls. This is achieved with a matrix retainer attached to a metal band and appropriate wedges, placed using tweezers, to contour the band, plus burnishing into shape with a hand instrument. This enables the amalgam to be effectively condensed and helps provide a contact point to avoid overhanging material and food packing.

The capsulated form contains a pre-measured alloy powder consisting largely of silver (61%) along with smaller amounts of copper (13%) and tin (26%). These percentages may vary with different amalgams and some may contain a small trace of zinc. The alloy also varies in the shape of the particles contained in the capsule. Some are lathe cut, spherical or a mixture of both. A pre-measured amount of mercury sealed within a membrane is also within the capsule. This membrane is broken during the mechanical mixing of the capsule (trituration) to allow the mercury and alloy to 'amalgamate'. The machine designed to mix amalgam is known as an amalgamator.

Capsule preparation sometimes requires a specially made device to activate the capsule, prior to trituration, to ensure that the mercury does mix with the alloy. Other types of capsule are self-activating and therefore can be placed straight into the amalgamator.

The capsules vary in the amount of amalgam that they contain. This amount is measured in milligrams or referred to as 'spills'. The larger the cavity, the larger the spill content of the capsule needed.

Mixing time varies depending on the make of the amalgamator. The time range can be between 7–12 seconds but even these times can vary. It is therefore a requirement to read the information sheet that accompanies the product before use. This ensures that the material is prepared and used correctly and the user is aware of potential hazards.

Working time for the **'medium set'** can be around **2 minutes**. This will include the time it takes for the DN to collect the material into the amalgam carrier, the dentist to insert it into the cavity and condense with the amalgam condenser. This process is repeated until the cavity is full.

Removal of the matrix band involves gently separating the band away from the material using a straight probe and any excess material is removed with the aspirator tip. The wedges are removed with tweezers followed by the band. The band may be cut with scissors to allow removal laterally from the contact area.

Carving time can also vary depending on the product and so the dentist has the choice of a fast, medium or slow set. As an average the **'medium set'** is just over **4 minutes**.

Checking the occlusion is achieved by the use of articulating paper. It is important to get this right as it could lead to stress on the periodontal ligaments, causing discomfort and maybe pain. If left, it could then ultimately lead to problems with the temporomandibular joint.

Finishing can be carried out at the next appointment with amalgam finishing burs, green stones and brown and green abrasive rubber polishing points (see Figure 7.4).

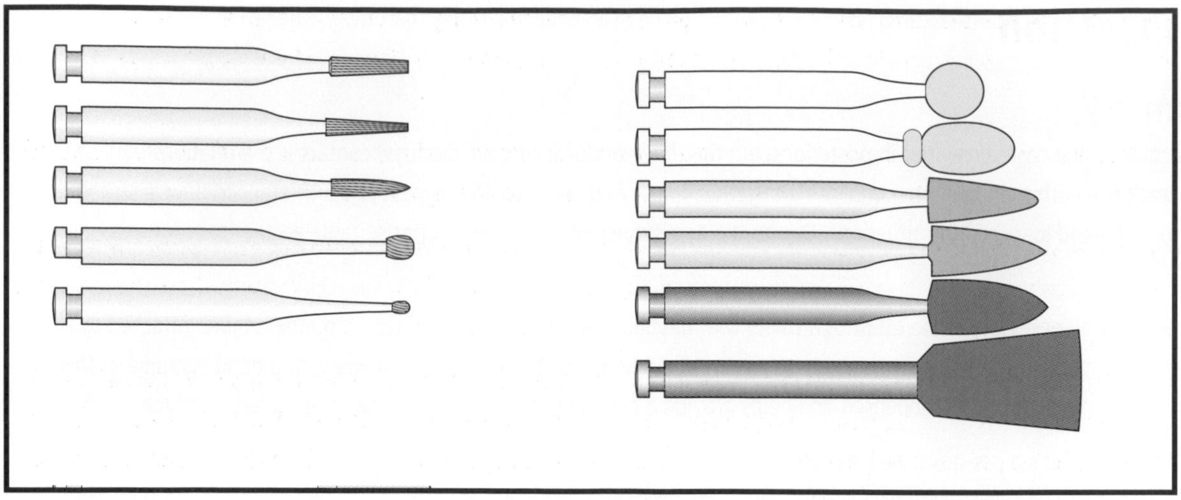

Figure 7.4: Finishing instruments burs including plain-cut steel finishing bars, stones, rubber points and abrasive rubber cup.

Safety issues

The mercury contained in amalgam is a toxic substance and is a risk to those handling it. Nowadays amalgam is available in capsule form and therefore the risk to dental staff is minimal. In spite of this, it is of the greatest importance to handle the substance with certain precautions (these will be mentioned later).

There seems to be no conclusive evidence supporting the idea that amalgam should not be used as a filling material, although there are occasions when the removal or placement of an amalgam filling is to avoided (e.g. patients who are pregnant). It may be decided that the placement of either a temporary filling or other satisfactory filling material is preferred.

Composite resin

The materials used to restore anterior teeth permanently are tooth coloured. Composite resins have been designed for this purpose because of their aesthetic qualities.

This group of materials has been developed over the years and there are many versions available. There are situations when composite resins are used to restore posterior teeth and the decision as to which material to use is made by the dentist, using the most appropriate material in each individual case.

Composite resins contain a resin and a filler. The filler may contain glass particles or quartz. The activation of the set may be chemical, for example, where an amount of Paste A (being the 'base') is mixed with an equal amount of Paste B (being the 'catalyst'). The working time that the dentist has with the 'chemically cured' composite is limited and so it is absolutely necessary for the dental nurse to prepare the material ready for the dentist to use without delay.

Other types of composite require exposure to a 'blue light' source to activate setting. This is known as 'light curing' composite. These materials give the dentist an increased working time compared to the chemically cured composite.

Some products are dispensed from a syringe and some are contained in a single-dose delivery tip, which is placed into a device for dispensing.

To enable the material to bond with the tooth and be retentive it is necessary to use a step-by-step bonding process using an acid etchant, primer, and bond system prior to the insertion of the composite filling material. An example of a light cured, delivery tip system is as follows:

Material shade needs to be selected, using the specific shade guide provided, before any treatment is undertaken. This ensures that the shade of the material matches the actual tooth. The tooth tends to lighten in shade while dehydrated and then darken to its normal shade when rehydrated.

Preparation involves the selection of the delivery tip and its insertion into the specialised dispensing device or applicator. The direction of the nozzle is adjusted depending on the position of the tooth cavity. This is carried out by the DN.

Matrix placement with wedges may be necessary to provide contact points, prevent overhangs and minimise the time taken at the finishing stage. The matrix needs to be transparent to enable the curing light to penetrate the material, otherwise the material will not set properly.

Cavity conditioning with an etchant gel containing around 36 per cent phosphoric acid is applied to the cavity surface and left for 15 seconds. It is then thoroughly rinsed for 15 seconds using the air/water syringe and aspirator tip. Some materials require the cavity to be dried gently without desiccation. The etching gives the tooth surface a white, frosty appearance. This will enable the composite to flow into the frosty surface and form 'tags', which aid retention.

It is important at this stage for the cavity to avoid the contamination of any excess moisture and saliva. This would be a procedure where the rubber dam would be of use.

Priming and bonding can be carried out either in two separate stages or combined, depending on the particular make. A drop of 'prime/bond' liquid is placed in a dappens pot and then applied to the tooth using a disposable brush tip. It is left on the tooth for 20 seconds. After this time the tooth is gently dried with the air/water syringe, ensuring that the water button is not inadvertently pressed. It is critical that the area is kept dry. The surface is then light cured for 10 seconds. It is necessary that the protective filter shield is used during the light curing process to ensure that the eyes of the dentist and DN are protected. The patient also needs to have suitable eye protection.

Placement of the composite restorative should be carried out immediately after the prime/bond stage. The DN removes the cap covering the nozzle and hands the applicator to the dentist who then squeezes the material into the cavity. The material is compacted into the cavity using a hand instrument such as a condenser. The cavity is filled in increments and these increments are light cured. The material is light cured for 20–40 seconds depending on the thickness of the increment.

Finishing can be carried out immediately after curing. Most of the excess, if there is any, can be removed using composite finishing burs or diamond burs. Fine finishing can be done using composite polishing strips and discs. Some manufacturers recommend special polishing pastes that can be used in conjunction with prophylaxis cups on a slow handpiece.

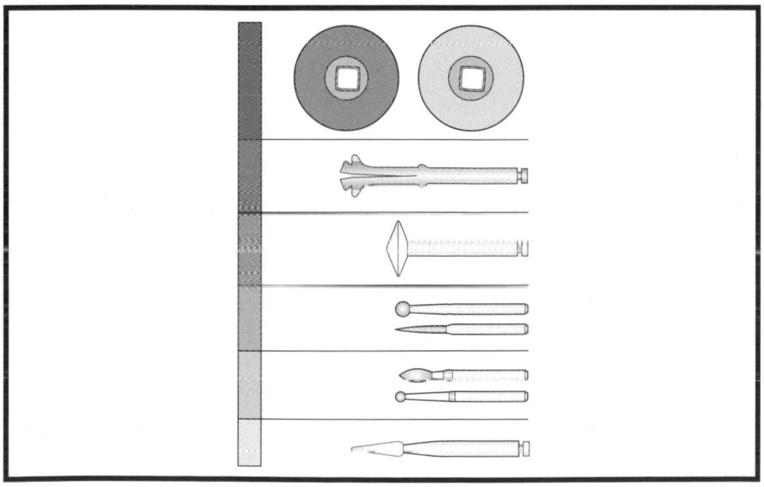

Figure 7.5: Composite finishing instruments e.g. strip, bars, mandrid and discs.

Glass ionomer

This material has been previously mentioned in the cavity lining section, but will also be mentioned in this section as it concerns permanent restorative materials.

Glass ionomers are tooth-coloured materials that are able to chemically bond to the hydroxyapatite in enamel and dentine. There are several types of glass ionomer cement with varying strengths. Some are designed for use in anterior teeth and some in posterior teeth. One example is a fast setting material that contains alumino silicate glass and polyacrylic acid. It is presented in powder form and is mixed with distilled or deionised water. This is a chemically cured material and it is essential for the dental nurse to mix the correct proportions of powder and liquid for the correct amount of time using a suitable mixing technique. This form of glass ionomer is suitable when permanently restoring the following cavities:

○ gingival cervical

○ approximal in an anterior tooth

○ a very small occlusal.

It is important to note that mixing techniques vary depending on the material. Although vigorous spatulation may be required for some materials it may not be appropriate for others!

Material shade should be chosen before the start of the procedure when the tooth is still hydrated. The next stage is to choose the items for matrix placement and to adjust them so that they will be ready to place as the material is inserted into the cavity.

Matrix placement for a gingival cervical cavity would need a soft metal matrix, which can be burnished to the correct contour using a hand instrument. In the case of an approximal cavity in an anterior tooth a transparent strip is used. Wedges may be used and, as mentioned before, this process contours the tooth to its original shape, reduces unnecessary excess, prevents overhang and saves time during the finishing stage.

The cavity should be washed and dried using an air/water syringe and aspirator tip prior to the matrix placement, otherwise the matrix may displace.

Cavity conditioning agents that are used prior to inserting a water-based glass ionomer contain 10% polyacrylic acid and are known as tooth cleansers. This is applied to the cavity for 15 seconds and then washed and gently dried with an air/water syringe and aspirator tip. The conditioner removes some of the dentine debris and the modified enamel surface known as the smear layer. This will aid the adhesion of the glass ionomer.

Mixing ratio is 1 scoop of powder to 1 scoop of liquid. This amount is increased in relation to the size of cavity (e.g. 2:2 or 3:3 etc).

○ Shake the powder bottle to mix up the contents then, using the scoop provided, place 2 level scoops of powder on the mixing pad provided or a cool glass slab. This amount would be enough for a medium size cavity.

○ Then completely invert the water bottle and by gently squeezing, place 2 drops of water onto the pad or slab, not too near the powder, otherwise it may combine with the powder before it is time to mix.

○ Using a stainless steel cement spatula, incorporate one of the scoops of powder with the water within 5 seconds or less, followed by the second scoop of powder in 10 seconds. It is important not to spend more than 20 seconds mixing as it is likely to break up the material during the chemical reaction. If this is allowed to happen then it affects the quality of the restoration.

○ The consistency of the end result should be like that of composite resin.

Working time from the start of the mix is 2 minutes. Setting time from the end of the mix is 2 to 3 minutes.

Placement of the material without the contamination of water and saliva relies very much on efficient moisture control using the methods already covered. The material is placed in the cavity in one increment and the chosen matrix is applied. The matrix should be kept in place for 4 minutes and as soon as the matrix is removed the restoration should be covered with a layer of light-cured bonding resin. This prevents the take up and loss of moisture, which may happen depending on the surrounding environment.

Finishing can take place at the next appointment although gross excess can be removed using finishing burs without water and then at the next visit finer finishing can be done using finishing strips, discs and specialised polishing paste with polishing cups.

Temporary restoration

Sometimes it is necessary to place a temporary restoration in a cavity in preference to a permanent one. Situations where this would arise include:

○ A tooth that requires a permanent restoration but may need monitoring.

○ Emergency treatment in the case of a fractured tooth or filling.

○ A convenient dressing in between the visits for root canal treatment.

○ Between the stage of a preparation and fit of a cast inlay.

Various materials for this purpose include the following:

○ zinc oxide and eugenol

○ glass ionomer

○ zinc phosphate.

Patient dismissal

At the completion of the treatment, the DN uses the air/water syringe and aspirator tip to rinse the mouth to remove any debris. When the patient feels that their mouth is comfortable, the chair is returned to the upright position. This may be done slowly if it has been a lengthy procedure and it avoids the patient feeling faint.

Instructions on aftercare are given to the patient and they in turn have an opportunity to ask any questions. A further appointment is made, if necessary.

Safe management of items after use

At the completion of the procedure it is important to dismantle sharp items carefully. The used disposable items that are sharp need to be placed in a 'sharps' container. These would include the local anaesthetic needle and anaesthetic cartridge. Metal matrix bands that have been in contact with amalgam are disposed of in a container especially for this purpose.

Other amalgam-contaminated waste includes the used amalgam capsules, the used dappens pot and the waste amalgam itself. There are also containers for these items that can be obtained from companies that specialise in this type of waste product. They arrange for collection and safe disposal.

Any other items that are not sharp, but that are disposable, are placed in a yellow clinical waste bag. This is collected along with the 'sharps' container by clinical waste contractors, and incinerated.

The usual cross infection control methods should be carried out for any other non-disposable item that has been contaminated. The surgery environment is then ready for the next procedure.

QUESTIONS

Question 2

a. Name three types of tooth wear.

b. What position should the patient chair be in for welcoming and consultation?

c. What position should the patient's chair be in for the procedure?

d. List the items needed for the protection of the dental team and patient.

e. What aspects of the operating field need to be controlled?

f. List the items needed for the control of the operating field.

g. What is the purpose of the aspirator tip?

h. Make a collection of manufacturers' mixing instructions and their material safety data sheets for the restorative materials mentioned in this chapter.

i. Practise mixing materials by carefully following manufacturers' instructions.

SECTION 3: Non-surgical endodontics Linked to DN21.1.2.3

Introduction

Treatments that involve non-surgical endodontics are pulp capping, pulpotomy and root canal treatment. These treatments are specific to the area of the tooth that contains the pulp tissue.

Pulp

This comprises nerve fibres, blood vessels, lymph tissue and connective tissue. The pulp tissue is surrounded by dentine in the centre of the tooth and is known as the pulp chamber. The root canal leads from this chamber to the apex of the tooth. The shape of the canal tapers and is very narrow at the apex of fully formed adult dentition. The opening from the apex of the tooth into the canal is known as the apical foramen and allows the blood and nerve supply to maintain the health of the pulp.

Cells known as odontoblasts are situated at the junction of the pulp wall and the dentine. These cells respond to stimulus and as a result they are capable of laying down secondary dentine. This response is for the purpose of protecting the pulp. Examples of stimuli include thermal, bacterial (caries) and chemical (calcium hydroxide cavity lining).

Some stimuli, such as thermal and bacteria, are so overwhelming that the odontoblasts are unable to lay down enough dentine to preserve the health of the pulp. Other cells found in the pulp are fibroblasts that produce collagen, which is the connective tissue that helps support the nerve, vascular and lymph tissues.

Pulp capping can be carried out if the damage to the pulp is repairable. This treatment enables the pulp to recover and, as well as restoring the function of the tooth, it preserves the vitality of the tooth. The pulpotomy procedure is covered in the chapter on Paediatric Dentistry.

Root canal treatment on permanent teeth is undertaken when the pulp is damaged irreversibly and there may be evidence of a periapical lesion. This treatment restores the function of the tooth and avoids extraction.

Situations where the pulp may become exposed, inflamed or necrotic include:

- deep caries
- over preparation of tooth with rotary instruments
- fracture of crown due to fall or a blow to the mouth.

To assess whether the pulp is in danger of being damaged or is already affected in some way, several methods for diagnosis are employed.

- Symptoms: the patient may have suffered discomfort and pain on eating foods that are hot, cold, or sweet. The longer the pain lasts, the more chance the pulp has disease.
- Tooth appearance: the dentist looks for caries and assesses its depth; and any abnormal discolouration.
- Special investigations: such as vitality testing and radiographs.

Vitality testing

In order for the dentist to make a diagnosis on the status of the pulp and then decide on appropriate treatment, it is beneficial to carry out a vitality test. The various methods for this diagnostic procedure involve stimulating the pulp by the introduction of **thermal** contact, **electricity** or **mechanical** contact.

Thermal – this can be a cold test using ethyl chloride which, whilst contained within a glass vial or pressurised canister, is in liquid form. It is sprayed onto a cotton wool pellet held by tweezers. The volatile liquid evaporates leaving an icy residue. It is then applied to a tooth that is known to be vital. This serves as a base-line response. The problem tooth is then tested. In all cases of vitality testing, it is important to explain to the patient that as soon as they feel a sensation they are to respond. Raising of the left hand is usually a pre-agreed sign. The dental nurse who then alerts the dentist can observe this response.

An example of a heat test is with the use of a very warm gutta percha stick. Vaseline may need to be used on the tooth surface prior to the contact of gutta percha to prevent it sticking.

Electricity – an electric pulp tester (EPT) is a battery-operated device that conducts a small electrical impulse to the pulp. To help in the conduction, a small amount of prophylaxis paste or Vaseline is placed on the tip that comes into contact with the tooth. There is sometimes an earthing plate, which needs to be in contact with the patient.

Mechanical – this involves starting a cavity preparation, with a bur and handpiece, without the use of a local anaesthetic. As soon as the patient feels a sensation the dentist will stop.

It is sometimes difficult for the dentist to interpret the results of a vitality test and so diagnosis may be difficult.

Pulp capping

There are two types of pulp capping.

Indirect pulp capping

This is carried out once the soft caries has been removed and the pulp has not been exposed. A layer of calcium hydroxide lining material is placed at the base of the cavity. This particular lining material is commonly used as it encourages the tooth to lay down secondary dentine and its alkaline content neutralises the acid formed by the bacteria. The bacteria become inactive in this adverse environment. The dentist then needs to assess whether the cavity requires an additional cavity base for strength and then a permanent restoration is placed.

Direct pulp capping

If the removal of caries has resulted in the exposure of the pulp then this is an indication that a direct pulp cap needs to be placed. All caries is removed and an assessment is made as to the level of contamination of the pulp. If the contamination is minimal then a layer of calcium hydroxide is placed over the exposed pulp and the restorative procedure continues as mentioned before.

In both indirect and direct pulp capping it is important that the patient is asked to monitor the tooth and take note if they have any further symptoms over a certain period of time. If there are symptoms then reassess.

Root canal treatment

The aim of this treatment is to remove the inflamed or necrotic pulp tissue, eradicate the bacterial contamination and fill the canal(s) permanently to prevent recontamination. This permanent filling of root canals is known as obturation. The anatomy of the root canal system can be very complex and incomplete obturation may lead to reinfection of the tooth.

There are many techniques that enable dentists to treat root canals and they include the use of manual files and specialised files that can be attached to a slow rotary handpiece and other mechanically or ultrasonic driven devices.

Surgery procedure

Preparation of the surgery environment

As with the dental procedures mentioned previously, the DN prepares the surgery by disinfecting work surfaces and setting out all the items required for that visit. The patients records and radiographs are made available.

Patient seating

The patient is greeted in the waiting area by the DN and escorted to the surgery where they are asked to sit in the dental chair safely and comfortably. The DN may need to adjust the chair to enable the patient to be seated and the headrest may also need adjustment.

The dentist consults with the patient regarding changes in medical history and any reports from the previous visit. The required treatment to be undertaken is discussed and, with mutual agreement, the treatment commences.

The DN informs the patient that the chair is to be placed in the supine position and a protective bib and eyewear is provided. The dentist and DN wash their hands, put on their eyewear, mask and gloves.

Control of the operating field

It may or may not be necessary to give local anaesthetic at this stage, as this would depend on the result of a previous vitality test. If it is evident that the tooth is responding to stimulus then a local anaesthetic needs to be given.

The rubber dam is applied by the dentist with the close support of the DN as mentioned in the section dealing with restorations. In the case of root canal treatment it may only be necessary to isolate the tooth being treated as this reduces the risk of the contamination of other teeth. This is not possible when treating a tooth that is the abutment of a bridge and therefore the whole bridge needs to be isolated. This is achieved by cutting slits between the holes that have been made in the rubber dam sheet. Isolation, in this case, is not ideal but it is a more sensible option than using no isolation at all.

If the rubber dam is difficult to apply, as the tooth is broken down, then it may be necessary to restore the tooth to enable the rubber dam to be applied. It is also necessary to ensure that the tooth is caries free before the start of root canal treatment. It is very important to use rubber dam when using small instruments and when using solutions containing sodium hypochlorite. In addition to retracting soft tissues, rubber dam prevents the inhalation or swallowing of small instruments and it protects the patient from swallowing any irrigating solutions. In addition, the use of rubber dam for endodontic procedures helps prevent the recontamination of the root canals during treatment.

If the patient finds it difficult to swallow once the dam has been applied then a disposable saliva ejector can be placed behind the rubber dam sheet in the floor of the mouth.

Canal preparation

Using handpieces and burs, access is gained to the pulp via a suitable surface. The DN removes the water and tooth debris using the aspirator tip.

A suitable tooth surface for:

❍ An upper anterior is *palatal*.

❍ A lower anterior is *lingual*.

❍ Premolars and molars is *occlusal*.

As mentioned earlier, there are various techniques of preparing root canals including:

❍ Step-back using hand files.

❍ Step-down using hand files.

❍ Step-down using rotary files.

QUESTIONS

? **Question 3**

Ask your dentist about the step-back and step-down techniques.

The DN has ready all endodontic items needed in the correct order for use and within easy reach of the dentist. Various stands for instrument presentation are available, or transfer using specialised tweezers may be preferred. The safe transfer of instruments can be done in the 'transfer zone', which is the area out of sight of the patient, a small distance away from the chin.

Apart from the instruments needing to be in the correct order, it is very important that they are the correct measurement.

Once access has been gained to the pulp all the coronal pulp tissue is removed to prevent coronal discolouration and the canal(s) are then located. At this point the air rotor and air/water syringe is not used as it is possible for the air and water used under pressure could damage the root canal.

Although we learn in tooth anatomy that each tooth has an expected number of roots, it is well known that these roots may have more than one root canal. Various names are given to these additional canals: accessory, lateral, loops and fins. Some of these canals can be treated effectively and some not.

Entry to the canals is initially made using an ISO (International Standard Organisation) size 08 or 10 file and enlarged to a certain extent. It is important to enlarge the opening of the canals so that the instruments can be inserted easily but without removing too much tooth tissue. Gates Glidden burs sizes 1 and 2 can also be used to enlarge the opening of the canal.

The next stage is to remove the pulp from the canal. This can be done using a barbed broach. The barbed broach is a 'single use' instrument, which is inserted into the canal and the tiny barbs on the end of the instrument engage in the pulp tissue and the pulp is removed from the canal on the withdrawal of the instrument. The canal may be irrigated using 1% sodium hypochlorite in an irrigating syringe. This solution has the advantage of dissolving organic substances and it also allows easy insertion of files (see Figure 7.6).

The DN should avoid any of the solution coming into contact with soft tissues or clothing.

The only accepted route of the sodium hypochlorite would be from the irrigating syringe into the root canal then into the aspirating tip!

A diagnostic X-ray is taken to determine the working length of the canal. A file is selected that will be wide enough to be seen easily on the radiograph. The file is measured to a pre-determined length using a periapical radiograph taken previously.

A measuring device known as an apex locator may be used. This determines the canal length using electrical conductivity. Although this may be time saving, it is important to have a radiograph for accuracy and a permanent record. Once the working length has been determined, the preparation of the canal(s) can be continued using a chosen technique.

Step-back involves starting with inserting the smallest size file measured to the working length into the canal, followed by the next size up and so on until a suitable size is reached e.g. size 30. As well as the removal of residual pulp tissue and contaminated dentine, the files are designed to shape the canal to receive the root canal filling. In between the change of file size, the canal is irrigated to help ensure the debris is removed. The DN can carefully remove the debris from the files, avoiding injury, using a gauze napkin that is damp with sodium hypochlorite.

Once a suitable size file has been reached e.g. size 30, with the step-back technique, the next size to be used is 35 but measured to 1 mm less than the previous file.

As the files increase in size, the length decreases by 1mm to shape the canal, irrigation removes debris and the return to the size 30 measured to the working length of 20mm (recapitulation) ensures that the debris is removed to the full length of the canal.

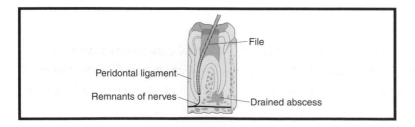

Figure 7.6: Position of endodontic file in root canal.

This procedure can be time consuming, but with the effective support of the DN in accurately measuring the instrument and providing a constant supply of irrigation, it can progress efficiently and save time.

Rotary instrumentation involves the placement of rubber dam, gaining access to the root canal as mentioned before and then using engine files in a specialised handpiece with a speed of 250 rpm, which can be adjusted. The instruments are used in a step-down technique and sodium hypochlorite is used for irrigation. Once the instrumentation is complete and the canal(s) are irrigated for the last time, they are then dried thoroughly using a cotton wool pellet followed by paper points. As the instrumentation is rotary it is a less time-consuming procedure. The DN measures and changes the files when needed and provides constant irrigation.

Some of the problems that may arise during canal preparation include:

- ledge forming during instrumentation
- perforation into periodontal ligament (lateral perforation)
- perforation through to the apex (apical perforation)
- perforation of a multi rooted tooth (furcation perforation)
- residual pulp tissue left in canal
- irrigating solution exuding through apex
- calcified blockage
- broken instrument.

Careful instrumentation and irrigation will avoid the problems mentioned above and a calcified root canal is usually cleared using EDTA (Ethylene Diamine Tetracetic Acid).

This can be introduced into the canal using a file or paper point. Perforations such as lateral perforations can be treated with the use of specialised slow setting calcium hydroxide for root canals. A layer is applied on the inner wall of the canal over the perforation using a file or rotary paste filler.

Temporary dressing

On the completion of the canal preparation, the canal(s) are irrigated and dried with a cotton wool pellet on tweezers to absorb most of the moisture, followed by paper points of a suitable size, also transferred on tweezers, to thoroughly dry the canals. The tooth, at this stage, will usually be dressed on a temporary basis and an interval of approximately a week will pass before the canals are filled permanently. If there is possible residual infection present, then an antiseptic medicament is placed in the pulp chamber on a small cotton wool pellet, or a form of calcium hydroxide can be placed down the canal(s). The tooth can then be temporised using a dressing material such as zinc oxide and eugenol.

The patient is advised to report any symptoms that they may have during the week to follow and to return if the temporary filling becomes displaced, as recontamination of the canal(s) may occur.

Permanent root filling (obturation)

At the next visit the tooth is opened under rubber dam, the temporary filling is removed and the canal(s) are reopened using the suitable size file measured to the working length. If there have been no symptoms since the last visit and there is clean, dry dentine on the file on reopening then the canal(s) are ready to fill permanently. The canal(s) are irrigated and then dried thoroughly with a cotton wool pellet followed by paper points passed on tweezers.

The DN prepares a suitable size gutta percha point (e.g. size 30) and a mark is placed at the working length. This *master point* is passed in tweezers to the dentist who then inserts it into the canal. This is to ensure it is an accurate fit. To enable easy insertion of a gutta percha point that may have become too flexible in a warm environment, it is sometimes helpful to place the gutta percha point on an alcohol wipe. This cools off the point and it is then easier to place in the canal. Once the dentist has tested the accuracy of the fit of the master point it is then ready for cementation. The DN mixes equal amounts of the root canal sealer paste's base and catalyst on glass slab of mixing pad, using a metal spatula, to a homogenous consistency. *The working and setting times for root canal sealers are usually quite lengthy. For instance, working time can be 4 hours and setting time can be 8 hours.*

This mix is presented to the dentist in the transfer zone along with the *master* gutta perch point in tweezers. The dentist dips the point in the root canal sealer and inserts it into the canal.

Sometimes the root canal sealer is placed into the canal using a rotary paste filler either used manually or in a slow speed contra angled handpiece. The DN takes back the tweezers and passes the finger spreader or thermal condenser. Once the master point has been condensed the DN passes accessory gutta percha points on tweezers, alternating with the condensing instrument, until the canal has been filled. Lack of effective condensing may lead to reinfection and therefore failure of the root filling. The excess gutta percha is removed and a temporary dressing of zinc oxide and eugenol is placed. The rubber dam is removed and a post operative X-ray is taken to ensure that the root canal filling has been placed correctly.

Patient dismissal

At the completion of the treatment, the DN uses the air/water syringe and aspirator tip to rinse the mouth to remove any debris. When the patient feels that their mouth is comfortable, the chair is returned to the upright position. This may be done slowly if it has been a lengthy procedure and it avoids the patient feeling faint.

Instructions on aftercare are given to the patient and they in turn have an opportunity to ask any questions. A further appointment is made, if necessary, for example a further appointment is made for the patient to attend for the permanent restoration.

The patient is again advised to report any symptoms that may occur from the time of the root filling placement to the time of the permanent restoration.

Safe management of items after use

As with all procedures, any disposable items are safely disposed of with special attention to sharp instruments such as barbed broaches. The effective cleaning and sterilising of root canal files has recently become a point of discussion due to Creutzfeldt-Jakob Disease (CJD) or the newly described 'variant CJD' (vCJD). It is one of a small number of human transmissible spongiform encephalopathies (TSEs) and it is believed that the disease may be transmitted by proteins, known as prions, that are present in pulps of infected individuals. The prions adhere to the root canal files and are impossible to remove. If they are present on the instruments when in the autoclave, their elimination is not guaranteed. With 'universal precautions' in mind it seems necessary to regard root canal instruments as disposable.

Question 4

a. Draw a labelled diagram of the tooth and its supporting structures.

b. Name the treatments that are regarded as non-surgical endodontic procedures.

c. What are the situations where the pulp may become exposed?

d. Name items needed for vitality testing.

e. What method is used for controlling the operating field during root canal treatment?

f. What can be done if the patient finds it difficult to swallow while the rubber dam is in place?

g. What is the name of the area where the safe transfer of instruments is carried out?

h. Where is the safe area for transfer of instruments situated?

i. What is the suitable size of endodontic file needed for the diagnostic radiograph?

j. What solution is prepared for the irrigation of root canals?

k. What is prepared to dry the canals?

l. Name the solution that dissolves calcium deposits in a root canal.

m. Name the materials used to permanently fill a root canal.

n. Give the reason why root canal files may need to be disposed of after treatment.

SECTION 4: Fixed prostheses Linked to DN20.2

Introduction

This section will cover the group of restorations that are formed out of the mouth and constructed on models in the laboratory of a dental technician. These are also known as cast restorations. These are permanently cemented restorations replacing the contour, function and anatomical shape (morphology) of the damaged part of the tooth. Restorations such as amalgam, composite and glass ionomer (which were mentioned in a previous section) are not cast but are called *plastic restorations*. *Plastic* in this case refers to the consistency of the filling material as it is inserted into the cavity. This consistency is easily pliable or mouldable.

Cast restorations to be covered in this section include:

○ Inlays

○ Veneers

○ Crowns

○ Bridges.

The use of cast restorations can be necessary for:

○ in the restoration of a weakened tooth to restore functional purposes

○ in aesthetic purposes in the case of a discoloured tooth

○ in the restoration of teeth with other forms of irregularity

○ in the restoration of a missing tooth or teeth

○ in occlusal rehabilitation.

A *plastic* restoration may be unsatisfactory due to the inadequate retention of the existing tooth structure. Missing teeth can be replaced by a fixed prosthesis known as a *bridge*. Functional purposes include the restoration of mastication and occlusion which, if not corrected, may lead to problems with the temporomandibular joint (TMJ).

Teeth can be replaced to improve the appearance (aesthetics) in the case of the anterior part of the mouth.

Inlay

This is an intra-coronal restoration that is cast outside the mouth and cemented permanently into the intra-coronal part of the tooth. The cavity must be prepared with no undercuts. This allows the cast restoration to be fitted in the cavity. Inlays can be cast in gold, composite and ceramic materials. A similar restoration with some occlusal coverage is known as an onlay.

Gold inlay

A gold inlay can be used when strength and durability are needed (see Figure 7.7). If it fits the cavity accurately and is cemented with an appropriate luting cement that is mixed well then it makes an excellent restoration. If it fails to fit accurately then there is a distinct possibility that the luting cement will dissolve. This leaves the tooth vulnerable to carious attack.

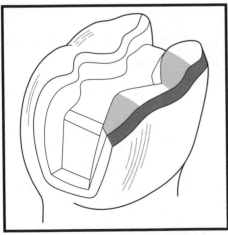

Figure 7.7: Tooth preparation of an MOD inlay with cuspal coverage (no undercuts).

Ceramic inlay

A ceramic inlay can be used when aesthetics is important. Some individuals prefer not to show any metal work when they smile or laugh. Some professionals such as singers or actors may opt for a tooth-coloured restoration.

The materials and laboratory techniques have been updated over the years and it is possible to construct a restoration that is reasonably durable.

Composite inlay

A composite inlay is a tooth-coloured restoration that can be constructed at the chairside or in a laboratory. It requires a curing oven and, if the construction is undertaken at the chairside, then this allows for any adjustments to be made immediately. Cementation is with a composite luting cement after the use of acid etch and bonding techniques. As with the ceramic inlay, the composite inlay is reasonably durable but for areas of the mouth that are load bearing the gold inlay would be more appropriate.

Veneer

A veneer is a tooth-coloured extra-coronal cast restoration that can be made in a ceramic material such as porcelain or in composite; and covers the labial surface of anterior teeth. It could be used in the case of discolouration. In the case of a minor irregularity such as a small diastema, two veneers could be used to close the gap. The tooth preparation is minimal and therefore regarded as less destructive than some cast restorations require. A composite luting cement is used to cement the veneer and the technique is similar to the cementation of a composite inlay.

Crown

A crown is the name given to an extra-coronal cast restoration that is permanently cemented and can cover three-quarters of the tooth surface or the entire tooth surface. A crown that covers all the surfaces of the tooth is known as a *full veneer crown* or *full coverage crown*. Crowns covering less than the full surface of the crown are known generally as *three-quarter crowns*.

The choice of crown would depend on the state of the tooth and its requirements, for example, whether the tooth is vital or non-vital. In the case of a non-vital tooth it would need to be root filled prior to the crowning. The crown would then need to be retained in the tooth with a cast post or retentive core of some sort. Another form of retention uses pins incorporated into the casting.

Choices of crown include:

○ Partial veneer. This can cover $3/4$ or $7/8$ of the tooth surface leaving the buccal or labial surface intact apart from a small amount of gold that will be visible. Tooth prepared with chamfer margins.

○ Full veneer metal. Used in the posterior part of the mouth where aesthetics is less important. There is little tooth preparation and the usual material used is gold. Tooth can be prepared with chamfer, knife-edge, shoulder or bevel margins.

○ Porcelain jacket. Usually used in the anterior part of the mouth where aesthetics is important. Not suitable for areas of the mouth that are load-bearing. Tooth can be prepared with shoulder margins.

○ High strength porcelain. Can be used in the posterior part of the mouth and uses up-to-date ceramic materials without the need for metal. Tooth can be prepared with a shoulder or chamfer.

○ Resin bonded porcelain. Used in the anterior part of the mouth for aesthetic purposes and tooth preparation is less destructive than in high strength porcelain crowns. Tooth can be prepared with a chamfer margin.

○ Porcelain bonded to metal. Can be used where strength and aesthetics is important. Tooth preparation involves removing substantial tooth tissue. Tooth can be prepared with a labial shoulder and lingual chamfer.

○ Composite crowns. A modern technique that can be used where aesthetics is important. Tooth can be prepared with a shoulder or chamfer.

Post and cores

As mentioned before, post and cores are used for the retention of crowns in teeth that have been root filled (see Figure 7.8). Types include cast, prefabricated and hybrid. The cast post and core is made in the laboratory. The prefabricated is made at the chairside using preformed posts and corresponding twist drills. The hybrid technique is a combination of the cast and prefabricated techniques. These options are carried out at the preparation and impression stage.

Amalgam or a resin core system are further options that can be used in certain circumstances as in the case of root filled or extensively restored vital posterior teeth. The tooth is restored, as it would be for a conventional filling. It is then prepared as for a conventional crown preparation.

Pins

Pins can be incorporated into a cast restoration when extra retention is needed. The preparation is carried out using specialised pin-hole drills. The holes are drilled in carefully chosen places to aid retention but at the same time, not to weaken the tooth structure. Corresponding plastic pins are placed into the holes at the impression taking stage and so, when the set impression is taken out of the mouth, the plastic pins are incorporated into the impression. This is sent off to the laboratory and the technician constructs a cast restoration with pins that fit exactly into the pin-holes. For an accurate fit, the pin-holes need to have been drilled parallel with each other, otherwise the finished article will not fit exactly.

Bridge

This is a fixed prosthesis that is permanently cemented to remaining teeth, replacing a missing tooth or teeth. There are bridges that are retained by implants that are fixed (see Figure 7.9).

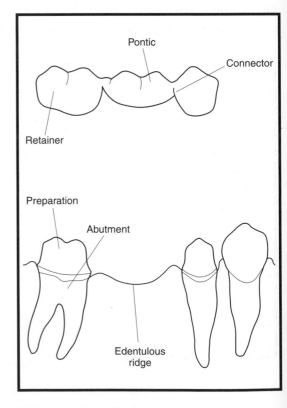

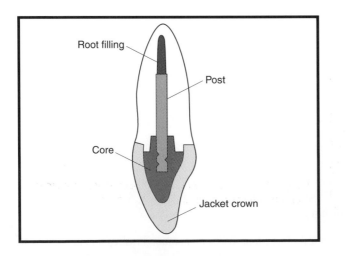

Figure 7.8: Prefabricated post with a cast core.

Figure 7.9: Components of a bridge.

Designs of conventional bridges include:

○ Fixed-fixed. Retainers and pontics joined together by rigid connectors. A common type used when abutment teeth are *not* tilted.

○ Fixed-movable. Rigid connector that joins a retainer with one side of the pontic. The other side of the pontic is joined to another retainer by a non-rigid connector. Used when abutment teeth *are* tilted (see Figure 7.10).

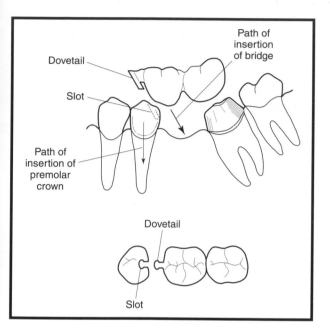

Figure 7.10: Fixed, movable bridge that can be cemented in sections for tiled teeth.

○ Cantilever. Retainer connected to only one side of the pontic leaving the other side unattached. This may be used if the tooth on one side of the pontic is sound. The use of an adhesive bridge may be an option (see Figure 7.11).

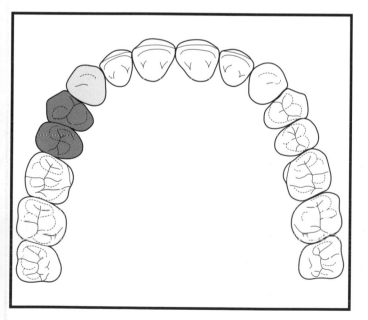

Figure 7.11: Cantilever bridge with upper right premolars as retainers and upper right canine as the pontic.

○ Spring cantilever. Retainer a distance away from the pontic connected by a metal bar. The retainer is usually in the posterior part of the mouth where the pontic is anterior. This design can be used if there are diastemata adjacent to the area of the missing tooth (edentulous area). The design may be difficult to keep clean as the metal bar embeds into the palate (see Figure 7.12).

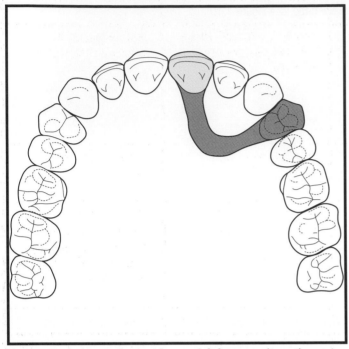

Figure 7.12: Spring cantilever with upper left first premolar as the retainer and the upper left incisor as the points joined together with a bar.

An **adhesive bridge** comprises retainers known as wings and they are connected to a pontic. The wings are cemented onto the abutment teeth with an adhesive resin. These bridges may have two wings or just one wing. Designs of early adhesive bridges included 'Rochette' which consisted of a pontic connected to wings that were perforated to aid retention. Another type is known as a 'Maryland' where the fitting surface of the wings was treated by 'electro-etching'.

These designs are now 25–30 years old and have now been superseded with types where the fitting surface of the wings is sand blasted to improve the quality of adhesion. These types presently used should be referred to as *resin retained bridges* or *adhesive bridges*. The tooth preparation for this type is minimal and requires little tooth destruction.

This technique is ideal to replace missing teeth in areas of the mouth that have sound or virtually sound teeth. It may not be acceptable to use designs that require much preparation of sound teeth.

Impression materials

Name	Use	Advantage	Disadvantage
Non-elastic materials			
Impression compound	Impression taking in areas with no undercuts. E.g. edentulous arches or tray modification. Available in cakes and sticks. Different colours denote different working temperatures.	Softening easily adjustable with temperature and reversed if necessary.	Not suitable in the presence of undercuts.
Impression waxes	Direct impressions of cast restoration preparations to produce a wax pattern.	Less laboratory time needed.	More surgery time needed.
Inlay pattern resin	Direct impression of cast restoration or as a combination method incorporated with an impression in a synthetic elastomer.	Added in increments to ensure accurate pattern.	Not suitable for undercuts (which should not be present anyway in the case of cast restorations).
Synthetic elastomers			
Polysulphide	Indirect impression. Now found only rarely.	Lengthy working time therefore an advantage if there is more than one preparation.	Messy to handle and has a similar odour to bad eggs! Lengthy setting time but can be accelerated with the addition of water at the mixing stage. Other materials are found to be more accurate.
Polyether	Indirect impressions and occlusal records.	Impression may still be usable if taken in conditions where moisture control is a problem. Setting time is less than 5 minutes.	May absorb water in storage from the environment and therefore distort. The set material is quite rigid and so not advisable for areas of marked undercuts as impression would be very difficult to remove.
Silicone	Two methods of setting (polymerisation). Commonly used impression material for cast restorations.		
– Condensation	Type I, condensation cured.	Good elastic properties. No unpleasant flavour.	Changes due to condensation requires the impression to be cast within 6 hours.

Name	Use	Advantage	Disadvantage
– Addition	Type II, addition cured.	The most stable of impression materials. Good elastic properties. No unpleasant flavour. Recent material (a polyvinyl) is able to take an accurate impression where moisture control is a problem.	Impression can be cast several days after being taken.
Hydrocolloids			
Reversible	Agar has been used for crown impressions in the past but there are other more appropriate materials to use.	Viscosity can be controlled by adjusting water temperature that flows through tray.	Requires specialised expensive equipment. Tears easily and a tendency to distort.
Irreversible	Alginate used for the casting of study models and opposing models in the construction of cast restorations.	Easy to use, inexpensive.	Once set viscosity is not changeable. Tears easily and a tendency to distort

Diagnosis and treatment planning

This is a very important stage and there is much for the dentist and patient to consider. If *plastic* restorations are inappropriate then cast restorations should be considered.

In the event of missing teeth, a decision needs to be made as to whether the space needs to be filled and if so, there is a choice to be made between removable prostheses and fixed prostheses. If the tooth has been recently extracted then it is necessary to wait for the alveolar bone to resorb. This may take up to three months. If a permanent bridge is placed in this area too soon after extraction then an unsightly gap is likely to appear under the pontic.

The patient's motivation and oral hygiene status are examined, as it is vital that the patient's oral hygiene is excellent. If it falls short of excellent then steps need to be taken to improve it or treatment options are reconsidered. It is not a good idea for this complex work to be undertaken in the presence of plaque!

Preparation of the surgery environment

The dental nurse sets out the required items for cast restorative procedures observing methods of cross infection control and efficient chairside assisting. Patient's records, radiographs and study models should be made available.

Patient seating

The patient is welcomed into the surgery by the DN where they are seated in the dental chair. The DN may need to adjust the height of the headrest for patient's comfort.

The dentist checks with the patient regarding changes in medical history and any reports from the previous visit. The required treatment to be undertaken is discussed and, with mutual agreement, the treatment commences.

The DN informs the patient that the chair is to be placed in the supine position and a protective bib and eyewear is provided. The dentist and DN wash their hands, put on their eyewear, mask and gloves.

Pre-tooth preparation

Items needed include:

○ Diagnostic and restorative instruments

○ Handpieces (air rotor high speed, contra angled slow speed and straight)

○ Burs and stones.

Method

If the tooth is vital, the dental nurse prepares the local anaesthetic (LA) syringe and places it within easy reach of the dentist. Due to the risk of needlestick injuries some dental teams do not transfer LA syringes directly into each other's hands but place them on a convenient surface where they can be resheathed safely.

Shade

While the local anaesthetic is taking effect, the shade can be taken at this point or left to the end of the procedure. The shade guide is held in the appropriate position in the mouth either in natural daylight or in an area that has good artificial lighting. The chosen shade is recorded in the notes and on the laboratory request form.

Tray selection

If a custom-made temporary is to be constructed then an impression can be taken prior to any tooth preparation. The DN selects two appropriate stock trays using study models (if available) to measure the correct size. One tray is used for the construction of the temporary and the other will be used for the taking of the master impression once the tooth or teeth have been prepared. The selected trays are handed to the dentist in order to try in the mouth. The impression material used for the purpose of the temporary construction may be alginate or sometimes a silicone putty is used. The appropriate adhesive is placed on the tray. Likewise, an appropriate adhesive is placed in the tray, which will be used for the master impression. This is put to one side and will be ready to use at a later stage. If a custom-made tray is preferred for the master impression then there are techniques available that enable a tray to be made in the surgery environment using a thermoplastic material. Tray adhesive can be placed on the tray at the beginning of the treatment session.

Initial impression for temporary

The DN prepares the impression material. In the case of **alginate**, the powder container is inverted several times to loosen the constituents and then level scoops are placed in the mixing bowl.

Some constituents of alginate include:

○ Diatomaceous earth

○ Potassium alginate

○ Calcium sulphate

○ Magnesium oxide

○ Colouring

○ Flavouring (peppermint oil).

☞ Alginates that contain peppermint oil should not be used on patients with allergies to peppermint oil.

Mixing ratio

When levelling the powder, be careful not to compress the powder into the scoop, as this will give an inaccurate measure. The number of scoops depends on the amount of material needed. For a sectional impression **1 level scoop powder to lower level of water measure**. An average size impression requires **2 level scoops powder to levels of water measure**. The consistency can be made thinner by increasing the amount of water and made thicker by decreasing the amount of water.

Mixing

○ The measured powder is placed into the rubber mixing bowl.

○ A well is made in the powder with an alginate spatula.

○ The measured water is added.

○ The powder is carefully, but rapidly, incorporated into the water and vigorously mixed within 30 seconds, ensuring that air bubbles have been dispelled as best as possible and a smooth mix is achieved.

Working time

○ After mixing, the DN places the mix into the tray with enough force to extrude some material through the perforations of the tray (if there are any).

○ Ensuring critical areas are filled without overloading.

○ With the water at room temperature the working time is $1^{1}/_{2}$ minutes.

The DN passes the filled tray in the 'transfer zone' so that the dentist can firmly take hold of the tray handle. The tray is inserted into the mouth and the patient is advised to breathe deeply through their nose, especially if it is an upper impression and the patient finds it unpleasant.

Setting time

With the impression at body temperature it will take about $2^{1}/_{4}$ minutes to set.

To increase the working and setting time the water temperature needs to be decreased and to decrease the working and setting time the water temperature needs to be increased.

To ensure the material is set the dentist can test any excess material in the mouth and the DN can test any excess that is left in the mixing bowl.

The impression is gently removed from the mouth. The DN can assist with the removal of the set impression by using the air/water syringe to break the vacuum seal in the upper anterior region. The aspirator tip is ready to remove any alginate debris in the mouth and a damp gauze napkin ready to remove any debris around the lips and face.

The dentist examines the impression and decides that it can be used for the construction of the temporary. The DN rinses it under a tap of cold running water to remove any saliva and debris. The impression is wrapped in a damp gauze napkin and put to one side ready for use when needed.

Impression material set-up

The DN prepares the master impression delivery system ready for use. Some are automatic mixing systems that use specialised syringes and cartridges. An example is a polyvinyl material, which is a silicone addition cured material. It consists of a light body and a heavy body material:

○ The light bodied cartridge is inserted into its impression gun.

○ The end of the cartridge is removed to reveal the openings of the base and catalyst.

○ The trigger of the impression gun is squeezed gently to 'bleed' the cartridge (this ensures that both base and catalyst are free flowing with no blockages).

○ A mixing tip and intraoral tip are attached to the opening of the cartridge.

○ The heavy bodied cartridge is inserted into the impression gun and the same steps are followed as with the light bodied material *but it is not necessary to place an intraoral tip on the heavy bodied cartridge.*

The shade taking, initial alginate impression and master impression preparation will only take a few minutes and once this is done the tooth or teeth will be anaesthetised enough to start their preparation.

Tooth preparation

Method

The dentist uses the air rotor handpiece and appropriate burs to prepare the tooth or teeth for a master impression. The DN uses the aspirator tip to keep the area clear of water and debris and also to retract the soft tissues as in the case of cavity preparation mentioned in a previous section.

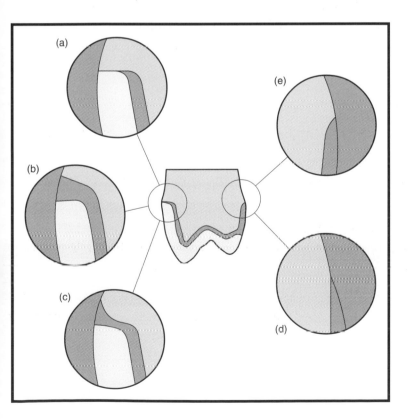

(a) Shoulder with porcelain butt fit;
(b) Deep chamfer with metal collar
(c) Shoulder plus chamfer (beval) with metal collar
(d) Knife edge with metal margin
(e) Chamfer with metal
Figure 7.13: Various tooth preparations.

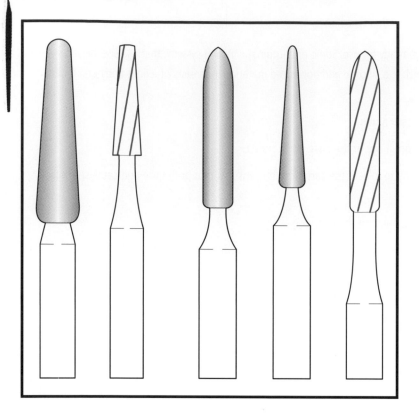

Figure 7.14: Burs used for preparations of full veneer crowns.

The preparation, of course varies, depending on the cast restoration to be made. The general rule for any cast restoration preparation is that it should be completely free of undercuts, as this will inhibit the path of insertion of the restoration. If there are unavoidable undercuts caused by caries then they can be blocked out with the use of a suitable filling material. Illustrations of different preparations can be found in this section (see Figs 7.13, 7.14).

Impression taking

There are two methods of impression taking:

❍ Indirect

❍ Direct.

The *indirect* method is covered later on in this section. The *direct* method can use blue inlay wax, which is placed on the tooth preparation and adjusted to the exact shape of the final restoration. The wax, which at this stage is known as a *wax pattern*, is carefully removed and sent to the laboratory where a cast restoration is constructed.

Items needed for impression taking include:

❍ Cotton wool rolls

❍ Dry guards

❍ Dry tips

❍ Cotton wool pellets

❍ Gauze napkins

- Gingival retraction cord

- Impression trays

- Impression material

- Tray adhesive

- Impression material accessories

  - Mixing receptacles

  - Mixing pads

  - Mixing spatulas

  - Syringes

- Impression disinfection solution and receptacle

- Sealable impression pouch with label

- Laboratory request form

- Impression transport box.

Method

This section covers impression taking using an indirect method using light and heavy bodied impression material.

- *If a post retained or pin retained crown is being prepared then preparation of the impression post or pins is undertaken at this stage and an appropriate impression post is 'tried-in', adhesive is applied to it and it is put to one side.*

- The DN passes a cotton wool roll to the dentist who then places it in the buccal sulcus in the area of the prepared tooth. If there is more than one tooth preparation then it may be necessary to place more than one cotton wool roll. These help keep the area dry and also retract the lip to a certain extent.

- The DN gently dries the area with an air/water syringe and passes a length of gingival retraction cord on tweezers to the dentist along with a flat plastic. The length of cord needs to be long enough to surround the tooth (see Figure 7.15).

- The dentist gently packs the cord into the sulcus of the gingiva. This sulcus is also known as the gingival crevice. The cord is designed to reduce gingival seepages and help to retract the gingiva away from the preparation. There are several other techniques that can be used to retract the **gingiva**, which include:

  - Electrosurgery – this is where a very fine metal tip is attached to a machine and it cauterises the gingival around the preparation. The cauterisation seals the gingiva and therefore reduces seepages. The machine should not be used in the near vicinity of an individual with a pacemaker as it may interfere with the pacemaker internal components.

  - Specialised paste containing an active ingredient of aluminium chloride can be placed in the gingival sulcus and left there for 1–2 minutes, after which it is rinsed leaving the area dry with the seepages under control.

  - Removal of soft tissue using a rotary instrument.

  - Application of a copper ring.

- The DN hands the dentist the tweezers for the removal of the retraction cord and the preparation is dried with the air/water syringe.

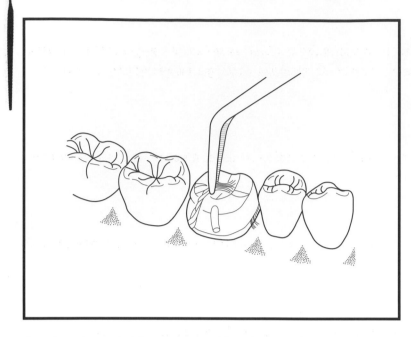

Figure 7.15: Removal of the retraction cord from the gingival sulcus.

○ The DN hands the pre-prepared syringe containing the light bodied material to the dentist. There is approximately $2\frac{1}{4}$ minutes of 'working time'.

○ *In the case of a post or pin retained crown, the temporary post or plastic pins need to be placed in the tooth preparation just prior to the 'injection' of the light bodied material.*

○ While the dentist syringes the light bodied material around the tooth or teeth preparations, the DN uses the syringe containing the heavy bodied material and fills the pre-prepared tray.

○ Tray containing the heavy bodied material is handed to the dentist once the light bodied syringe has been finished with and handed back to the DN.

○ The dentist inserts the tray into the mouth, shortly after placement of the tray the DN hands over the tweezers to remove the cotton wool roll(s). The pressure of the heavy bodied material directs the light bodied material further into the gingival sulcus. This action should create an accurate impression of the preparation(s).

○ While the material is setting, the DN ensures that the patient is as comfortable as possible. If there is any saliva collected at the back of the mouth it can be removed using the aspirating tip and being careful not to dislodge the impression and not to aspirate any setting material, as this may block the tip.

○ After approximately four minutes the material is set and the impression tray can be removed by the dentist.

Occlusal registration

Method

Occlusal registration is taken so that the technicians constructing the cast restorations in the laboratory have an accurate record of how the patient bites together. This then ensures that the finished article will fit the tooth or teeth accurately and not interfere with the way the patient bites together.

Pink wax

Occlusal registration can be recorded using pink wax that has been softened by the DN in warm water. It is shaped and then the dentist places it in the mouth so that the patient can gently bite into it. The DN can speed up the cooling of the wax with the use of air from the air/water syringe.

Bite registration paste

Some bite registration materials have the same delivery system as the impression materials and so it is a simple matter just to replace the impression cartridge with the bite registration cartridge.

Opposing impression

This is taken in alginate using the method of alginate impression taking mentioned before. This impression is then sent to the laboratory along with the other occlusal records.

Face bow

This record will help replicate the movement of the upper and lower dentition in relation to the temperomandibular joint.

○ The DN hands the face bow fork with softened wax to the dentist who places it in the patient's mouth.

○ The face bow itself is then handed to the dentist who places it onto the bite fork.

○ If using a Denar face bow, the ear lugs are then positioned in the ears and the reference plane locator is pointed towards the nose.

○ While the dentist positions the face bow components, the DN supports the main body of the face bow and when ready the DN tightens the locking devices.

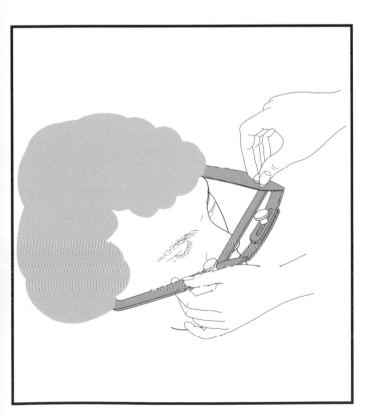

Figure 7.16: Positioning of the face bow.

Construction and cementation of temporary restoration

The purpose of temporising the tooth preparations is as follows:

○ Protect the tooth preparation against sensitivity of the pulp and damage.

○ Aesthetic purposes.

○ Functional purposes, but unable to withstand heavy loads.

○ To maintain space that ensures that the permanent restoration will fit accurately.

Items

○ Alginate and associated equipment.

○ Crown and bridge material.

○ Pre-formed crowns.

○ Temporary restoration cement.

○ Dental floss.

○ Articulating paper and forceps.

Method

○ Using the alginate impression taken prior to treatment, the DN mixes the temporary crown material and places it in the dispensing syringe.

○ The syringe and impression are then handed to the dentist who extrudes the temporary crown material into the imprint of the impression and repositions it in the patient's mouth.

○ The DN and dentist need to carefully monitor the setting reaction of the material, as there is a danger that the temporary crown material may shrink onto the tooth preparation if left on for too long. This is time consuming and a little frustrating for all concerned.

○ Once the material has reached its initial set, the dentist removes the impression and then removes the temporary crown material.

○ The excess material is removed from the temporary crown using a straight handpiece and suitable bur.

○ The modified crown is replaced in the mouth to test the fit and the occlusion using articulating paper on forceps, which is then handed to the dentist by the DN.

○ Once the fit and occlusions are correct the DN mixes equal amounts of the temporary crown cement on a pad using a cement spatula.

○ The DN places the cement in the crown using a flat plastic and passes the crown to the dentist who then inserts it onto the appropriate tooth preparations.

○ Once the cement has set the DN passes the straight probe or excavator to the dentist so that the excess cement can be removed.

○ The DN uses the aspirator tip to remove the debris.

○ The DN then passes a length of floss to the dentist who flosses around the temporary crown and the DN aspirates any further debris.

○ A final rinse using the air/water syringe and aspirating tip ensures the patient's comfort and they are then ready to be dismissed.

○ Instructions are given verbally to the patient by the dentist regarding the care of the temporary crown. The patient needs to eat carefully eat and gently brush around the area, as it is important to keep the gingival healthy. If the crown comes off then contact the surgery as soon as possible so that it can be recemented.

Fit and cementation of permanent cast restoration

Items needed:

○ Gauze napkins.

○ Specialised finishing burs (if necessary).

○ Dental floss.

○ Articulating paper.

○ Permanent cementation material.

  – Mixing pad or glass slab

  – Mixing spatula.

Method

○ Unless the dentist thinks that the patient will not feel much sensitivity during the fit and cementation, a local anaesthetic will be needed.

○ The DN hands the dentist a gauze napkin to protect the airway during the removal of the temporary crown, followed by an excavator to actually remove the crown.

○ The DN receives the temporary crown and then rinses and dries the preparation using the air/water syringe (being aware of possible sensitivity) while the dentist continues to use the excavator to remove any residual cement.

○ The DN carefully hands the permanent cast restoration to the dentist and it is then placed on the tooth or teeth preparations, still with the gauze napkin in place to protect the airway.

As well as the danger of the patient inhaling the restoration it is possible that the patient may accidentally swallow it. If it does somehow disappear down the back of the patient's throat it may be necessary to obtain radiographs. This locates the position of the restoration. Hopefully, the item had not been inhaled and if in the digestive tract, it will be only a matter of time before it can be retrieved!

○ Once the restoration is in place, the DN hands the dentist a straight probe, used to ensure the margins are well fitting.

○ To test the contact points are satisfactory the DN hands a length of dental floss to the dentist. It may be necessary for a finger to be placed on the top of the restoration to prevent it from coming away from the preparation.

○ The DN then hands articulating paper in forceps to the dentist who tests the occlusion by asking the patient to gently close together.

○ Any adjustments can be made out of the mouth using specialised burs on handpieces. With an excellent preparation, impression temporary restoration and laboratory support adjustment can be minimal if needed at all.

○ When the dentist and patient agree that the restoration is fitting well, it is then ready for permanent cementation.

- Cotton wool rolls are placed around the preparation and the area is gently dried using the air/water syringe.

- The DN selects the luting cement, measuring scoop, mixing pad and spatula. A glass ionomer has been chosen in this case but there are many other options for many situations.

- The bottle of powder is inverted several times to loosen the particles and an appropriate number of level scoops of powder are placed onto the mixing pad. The amount depends on the size or number of restorations or the number of units incorporated into a bridge.

- The mixing proportion is 2 scoops to 2 drops of water.

- The DN incorporates the powder into the water within 20 seconds and then loads the material into the fitting surfaces of the cast restoration using a flat plastic or spatula.

- The restoration is then handed to the dentist in a way that the dentist can easily orientate it for correct seating on the preparation.

- Once the restoration is seated, the dentist applies gentle pressure while the cement is setting.

- A straight probe or excavator is handed over and used to remove any excess cement once set and floss is used to clear debris interdentally.

- The dentist removes the cotton wool rolls, but if they are dry the DN needs to moisten them with water from the air/water syringe. This prevents damage to the oral mucosa on removal.

- There is a final rinse with the air/water syringe and aspirator tip and the patient's chair is returned to the upright position.

- Instructions are given to the patient regarding keeping the area clean and the patient has the opportunity to clarify any points.

- Apart from the usual toothbrushing, and floss, it may be necessary to recommend other methods of interdental cleaning and, in the case of bridges, floss threaders are recommended.

Laboratory communication

The technical staff have an important part to play in these procedures and it is therefore critical that the DN ensures that all impressions and bite registrations are sent intact and safely to the laboratory accompanied with a completed laboratory request form containing the vital information. The DN also discusses with the technical staff as to when the patient's appointments may be booked. This communication avoids the situation of the patient attending the surgery expecting a crown to be cemented and the DN having to explain to the patient that the crown is unfinished and is still at the laboratory.

The techniques available in laboratories vary from 'tried and tested' to 'up-to date' techniques such as digital shade taking and digital scanning of models.

Patient dismissal

As mentioned previously, at the completion of the treatment, the DN uses the air/water syringe and aspirator tip to rinse the mouth to remove any debris. When the patient feels that their mouth is comfortable, the chair is returned to the upright position. This may be done slowly if it has been a lengthy procedure and it avoids the patient feeling faint.

Instructions on aftercare are given to the patient and they in turn have an opportunity to ask any questions.

Safe management of items after use

Cleaning and disinfecting

It is recommended that impressions are disinfected prior to being sent off to a laboratory.

○ The dentist examines the impressions and bite registrations.

○ Decides that they can be used for (i) the construction of the permanent cast restoration and (ii) occlusal record.

○ The DN rinses them under the tap of cold running water to remove any saliva and debris.

○ They are then placed in a receptacle containing disinfecting solution suitable for impressions. These solutions are usually recommended by the manufacturers of impression materials.

○ Left in for the recommended time.

○ Remove and rinse thoroughly under cold running water.

○ The alginate impression is wrapped in a damp gauze napkin.

○ Place each impression and bite record in a separate sealable impression bag.

○ Label stating patient's name, practice name, date and time of disinfecting.

○ All items placed safely into a padded box for transport to the laboratory.

The surgery is cleared and prepared for the next procedure as mentioned in previous sections.

☞ Conclusion

For a dental surgery to run smoothly, it is essential that the DN has the knowledge of all aspects of dentistry including a detailed knowledge of dental procedures. Apart from knowledge, it is necessary to acquire the skill to put this knowledge into practice along with the use of initiative. An efficient and effective DN anticipates the needs of the dentist and patient.

In order to constantly improve good practice, it is advisable to keep up-to-date with new techniques. This can be achieved by attending relevant courses, gaining information from dental websites including dental company websites, reading dental text books and dental periodicals.

QUESTIONS

?

Question 5

a. State five reasons for restoring teeth with fixed prostheses.

b. Name a cast restoration that is cemented intracoronally.

c. Is a post and core necessary for a vital or non-vital, root filled tooth?

d. Name the components of a conventional bridge.

e. What is the material usually used to take the primary impressions for study models?

f. Is alginate a reversible or irreversible hydrocolloid?

g. If a patient has a 'gag reflex', what is important to remember when loading an impression tray?

h. What are the two methods of impression taking for cast restorations?

i. Which of the above methods takes up the most surgery time?

j. Which instrument is passed by the DN for the insertion of the gingival retraction cord?

k. What is a contra-indication for the use of electrosurgery?

l. State the reasons for placing a temporary crown on a prepared tooth/teeth.

m. Is a luting cement mixed to a creamy or putty consistency for the cementation of cast restorations?

n. List the items that need to be sent to the laboratory for the construction of a cast restoration?

References

Essentials of Dental Caries, The Disease and its Management Kidd EAM and Joyston-Bechal, S. (Oxford University press)

Pickard's Manual of Operative Dentistry Kidd, EAM and Smith BGN (Oxford University press)

Team Dentists: Chairside Procedures and practice management J Ellis Paul (Martin Dunitz)

Restorative Dentistry: An integrated approach Peter Jacobsen (Wright)

The treatment options to restore a space in the dentition are:

○   nothing

○   a denture

○   a bridge

○   an implant.

In crude terms, an implant is like a inserting rawl plug into the jawbone onto which a crown, denture or bridge can be placed. Dental implants have been used successfully for about 30 years and are made of titanium, which fuses to the bone, creating a very solid base for a prosthesis.

☞ The procedure takes place under local or general anaesthesia and because it involves surgery must be carried out under sterile conditions to prevent cross infection.

Once the implants are placed in the bone they must be left *in situ* for a period of three months in the mandible and six months in the maxilla. During this time the bone will attach to the implants, this is a process called osseointegration. When the implants have fully integrated and are stable, a prosthesis can then be attached.

Where teeth have been extracted, it is advisable to leave the site to heal for at least three months before placing implants.

Procedure

Consultation appointment

Many factors can affect the outcome of dental implants. X-rays or scans can be used to assess the thickness and quality of the bone. The position of the inferior dental nerve in the mandible must also be taken into consideration to prevent paralysis. If a patient is diabetic the healing can be affected and smoking is also known to reduce the success rate of implants by roughly 30 per cent. The dental nurse (DN) should ensure that a medical history form is completed by the patient. If the patient is taking aspirin or Warfarin the operator must assess whether this should be stopped before embarking on surgery.

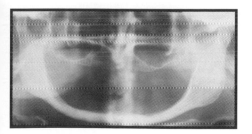
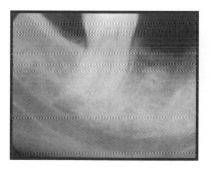

Figure 8.1 and Figure 8.2: OPG showing the inferior dental nerve and a periapical radiograph showing space for a single tooth implant.

☞ The DN should make sure that patients requiring antibiotic cover and have this arranged before the surgical appointments.

Stage I Surgery

This is when the implants are placed in the bone. The DN should ensure that the X-rays and patient notes are available and any relevant medical history is brought to the attention of the operator. When surgery takes place it is best to have two or three DNs assisting.

☞

○ DN 1 will pass the instruments to the operator.

○ DN 2 will irrigate and aspirate.

○ DN 3 will be on hand to open any packets or pass equipment needed throughout the surgery.

Obviously this is not always practical and you will have to adapt to the situation in your workplace.

All surfaces in the surgery must be washed down and prepared with suitable disinfectant. Attention should be paid to areas higher than eye level, which gather dust.

Instruments and equipment

When the equipment/instruments are being set up the DN should wear:

○ Mask

○ Surgical cap

○ Sterile gloves.

☞ Once sterile gloves are on only sterile items must be touched.

There are two sections to the implant instrument tray: titanium and stainless steel. The components made of each material should be kept separate by placing them in the allotted sections. DN 2 or 3 should open packets and drop any items onto the sterile drape in order for DN 1 to set up as shown. The DNs and the dental surgeon should plan for surgery by making sure all fixtures, tools and cover screws that are to be used are available in advance. It is important to check that all instruments are sterile and ready to be used.

☞ Before the procedure the DN can administer 3 gm Amoxycillin, or if the patient is allergic, an alternative can be given under instruction from the dental surgeon. This is to prevent infection. A painkiller can also be given before the surgery to ease any post-operative pain.

The patient is given a local anaesthetic, a cap and some safety glasses to wear. The operator and two DNs prepare for surgery by putting on a cap and mask, scrubbing hands and then putting on a sterile gown and gloves. The patient is covered with a sterile drape, the patient's mouth is wiped with a chlorhexidene solution and more local anaesthetic is given.

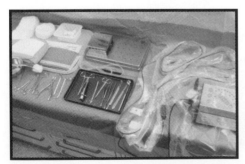

Figure 8.3: Instruments and equipment.

The operator makes an incision and the gingival tissue is lifted, exposing the bone. A surgical stent or a pencil may be used to show the position in which the implants will be placed. The operator will prepare the site for placement of the implants by using a sequence of drills. The site is measured and an implant of the appropriate length is chosen. The implant is inserted with a handpiece, set at 27 revs/minute. Copious irrigation is essential throughout the drilling period and when fixture is being installed, this is to prevent the bone from overheating, which can cause implant failure. The implant is then tightened by hand using a cylinder wrench. If a mount was used, this is now removed and a cover screw is placed on the implant to protect the internal aspect of the implant, the gingiva is then sutured back into position. The patient is then asked to apply pressure to the area by biting down on a sterile gauze to reduce the risk of haemotoma.

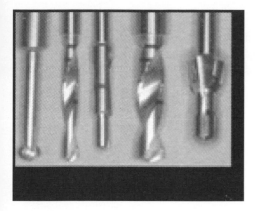

Figure 8.4: Sequence of drills.

All labels from components used should be kept in the patient notes for reference.

Post-operative instructions

The patient is given a course of antibiotics and a chlorhexidene mouthwash to be used twice daily for a week. A pain reliever can also be given to be taken the same evening. The patient is warned that they could experience some swelling and/or bruising, but this does not affect everyone. If the site bleeds a pack should be placed over the area and pressure applied. Most people are well enough to return to work the day following surgery.

The patient has to return to the surgery approximately one week later to have the sutures removed and for the operator to review their condition.

☞ After Stage I surgery it is important for the DN to distinguish between titanium instruments and stainless steel instruments. They should be kept separate throughout cleaning. All instruments should be placed in the ultrasonic cleaner, rinsed, dried thoroughly and then placed in packets for re-sterilisation. The handpiece should be oiled before being placed in a packet for re-sterilisation. If the handpiece separates this should be done before sterilisation.

Stage II surgery

After a period of healing has taken place, Stage II surgery can be performed. This is also carried out under sterile conditions but is a much simpler and less complicated procedure requiring fewer instruments.

The cover screw is exposed using a soft tissue punch, or a small incision is made. The cover screw is removed and a selected healing abutment is placed on the implant. If necessary the soft tissue is sutured around the healing abutment. Healing abutments are left in place for about 1–2 weeks, during which time the gingival tissue will heal around the abutment.

Abutment connection

At this appointment the healing abutment is removed and a definitive abutment is selected. The abutment used depends on the number and position of the implants. This will be decided by the operator. Healing caps are then placed on the abutments.

The following appointments will vary depending on the type of prostnesis to be used.

Prosthetic appointments

Single tooth implant

An impression coping is placed on the abutment and an impression is taken. An opposing impression is also taken to determine the position of the opposing teeth and the shade of the teeth is recorded. When the crown is ready it is fitted onto the abutment using a small amount of temporary cement. The bite and fit are checked.

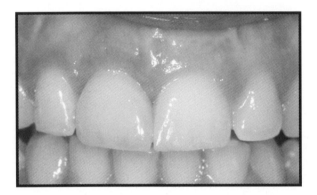

Figure 8.5: Single tooth implant with crown.

Implant retained fixed bridge

Appointment 1

Impression copings are placed onto the implants. The tray is prepared by removing plastic from the area where the impression copings protrude through. An impression is taken removing any material from the impression coping screws. The screws are undone and the impression is removed. An opposing alginate impression is also taken.

Appointment 2

One week later. The patient's bite is recorded using a customised base prepared by the laboratory.

Appointment 3

Two weeks later. The framework is tried in to check the fit, and the shade of the teeth is taken. It can be helpful if the patient can provide a photograph of the natural teeth at this appointment.

Appointment 4

The framework and the teeth set in wax are tried in the mouth. This is shown to the patient and if they are not happy with the appearance changes should be made at this stage.

Appointment 5

The prosthesis is fitted. The shade and fit are thoroughly checked and the access holes are filled with a plastic material, which can easily be removed for access at a later date by the operator.

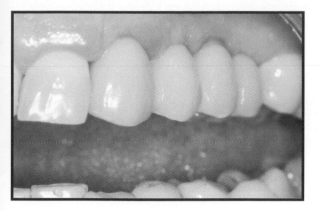

Figure 8.6: Implant retained fixed bridge.

Implant retained denture

Appointment 1

An impression is taken is exactly the same way as for a fixed bridge.

Appointment 2

A wax block, which is provided by the laboratory, is attached to the implants, and the patient's bite is recorded.

Appointment 3

A metal bar is provided by the laboratory. This is tried in by attaching it to the dental implants as shown.

Appointment 4

Teeth are set in wax and are shown to the patient. If the patient is not happy with the appearance it should be changed at this appointment.

Appointment 5

The denture is provided by the laboratory. The metal bar is fitted to the implants and the denture is clipped into place. The bite and fit are checked.

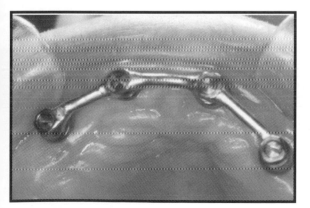

Figure 8.7: Implant retained denture.

☞ Post-operative care and cleaning

The patient is advised to clean their new prosthesis as they would their natural teeth. This includes flossing and general brushing. Plastic-coated interdental brushes can be used if needed. The patient should continue to see the hygienist as normal. The hygienist will use Teflon-coated or plastic-coated scalers and the patient is advised not to use woodsticks. In a patient's lifetime the prosthesis may need to be changed due to wear and general ageing. This can easily be done by following the procedure as before.

QUESTIONS

?

Question 1

a. What length of time should be left from extraction to implant placement?

b. What two factors can affect the outcome of dental implants?

c. Why is it important to use irrigation during drilling and fixture placement?

d. Name the two sections of a fixture installation box. What precautions should be taken regarding these?

e. How many prosthetic appointments are needed for

○ A single tooth implant

○ An implant retained fixed bridge

○ An implant retained denture?

PAEDIATRIC DENTISTRY

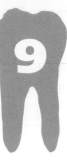

Introduction

This chapter is linked to DN12:1.2, DN15.3 and DN21.2 of the NVQ Level 3 in Oral Health Care. The aim of this chapter is to discuss and explore paediatric dental care, with regard to prevention, pulpotomies and traumatised permanent incisors. Each area of dentistry requires specific skills and various demands are made upon the dental team. In paediatric dentistry the dental visit will create a lasting impression on the child and it is up to the dental team to ensure that the experience is a positive memory. A child who develops a trusting and co-operative relationship with the dental team will remain a regular attendee for life. We are in the privileged position of introducing the child and quite possibly the family to an essential aspect of healthcare. Dental visits made during a child's formative years are therefore the foundations for the dental habits of the future adult. This makes involvement in paediatric care full of interest, rewarding and unique.

The environment

How do children see the dental surgery? Is it inviting and reassuring? What questions are they asking themselves? What does this machine do? What does that feel like? Why does that machine make a noise? What does that taste like? Will that hurt me? Is that something I can play with? Who is going to entertain me while my carer is answering questions? What am I allowed to touch? Why can't I touch this? Why do I have to sit still? Can I go now?

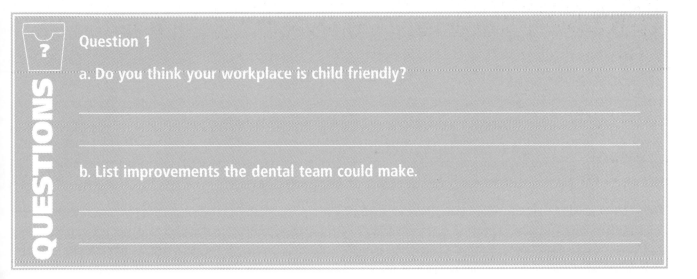

QUESTIONS

Question 1

a. Do you think your workplace is child friendly?

_____

_____

b. List improvements the dental team could make.

_____

_____

When preparing the surgery for the child patient, consider putting away all items not required. This gives the child less to worry about, makes the room seem less intimidating and offers fewer distractions. They do not realise that not everything on display will be used. Children are naturally restless and are unused to sitting still for long periods of time. Try to keep the appointments relatively short and prepare the surgery before they come in. Make sure that all instruments and materials likely to be used are close at hand. The less moving around that has to be done to locate things during the treatment will ensure the appointment is on schedule and will reassure and stop the child from moving around on the dental chair. A child who constantly has to be resettled by the dentist will feel uncomfortable, bored and 'restrained'. This can lead to frustration and, from their perspective, becomes an unpleasant visit. There is a limit to the working time available and it is imperative that the dental nurse (DN) can respond to and anticipate the dentist's needs promptly.

Six hands are a useful attribute for the DN, when the dentist is trying to place a restoration on a two-foot-two patient who is either sliding down the chair away from the dentist and the dental light, or has been able to turn their body into a corkscrew at a moment's notice!

Why bother?

Parental opinion will vary, usually as a direct result of their own experiences. It is possible that the adult may find it difficult to be in the dental surgery if they have experienced traumatic episodes as patients themselves.

The effort of multiple visits to restore the teeth may be seen as a waste of time. Arguments may include the following:

○   The primary dentition will fall out naturally at some point and be replaced.

○   If the child suffers pain the teeth can be taken out.

○   The adult may have difficulty taking time off work to bring the child.

○   The expense of travelling to the surgery may be a concern.

○   Childcare commitments for siblings can be an issue.

During the initial check-up visit it is important that a thorough history is obtained and an opportunity for discussion is available. Many issues can be addressed that may make planning a course of action beneficial to all parties. Regular screening can eliminate or reduce the amount of treatment required. The worst case scenario is to meet a child who is in pain and distressed and who will, through the adult carer, attend the surgery as an emergency case throughout their childhood. Remember: the child does not have an option. They cannot make choices for themselves, they rely on the adult to make the appointment and bring them to the surgery.

Implications

Premature loss of deciduous dentition can cause long-term difficulties. As children are going through an ongoing loss of teeth naturally, gaps are not unusual. However, removal of upper anteriors at the age of three due to 'bottle caries' can affect the development of speech. The tongue is unable to make contact with the palatal aspect of the centrals and certain sounds can become distorted, for example 'th'. The soft tissue of the gingivae will become hardened through eating and eruption of the permanent teeth can be delayed, which in turn can lead to drifting of the arch and insufficient room for other teeth to erupt.

If good dental habits are not established that include, amongst other things, regular check-ups, dietary advice and oral hygiene, the prognosis for a healthy permanent dentition is not favourable. Primary teeth that become grossly carious and have to be extracted when they become symptomatic will usually lead to orthodontic concerns in the future. remember **'PREVENTION IS BETTER THAN CURE'**.

Question 2

Is it likely that a patient who attends for emergency treatment is a good prospective candidate for orthodontic care? Discuss with your dentist.

QUESTIONS ?

_____

_____

_____

_____

The importance of giving appropriate diet advice

The dental team must look at the whole family group, including grandparents and friends, who will often regularly give children sweets, which, although well-meaning, can have an adverse effect on the child's teeth. Cultural differences are another factor, which if not taken into consideration can cause misunderstanding.

Some medical conditions require the child to take medication in the form of syrup medicine. Obviously the medical condition supersedes the dental needs, although this may have an effect on the child's teeth. Don't forget, there are often sugar-free alternatives.

The diet sheet

The diet sheet should incorporate two weekdays and a weekend day, as the majority of people eat differently at the weekend.

Question 3

Make a diet sheet specifically for a child and complete it yourself. You may find it interesting!

QUESTIONS ?

_____

_____

_____

_____

Encourage the child/parent/guardian to give honest answers, we want to give the best advice for their child, which will have a positive effect, if adhered to. Encourage sweet eating after a meal or on a particular evening. Suggest that when people give them sweets, they be put in a cupboard out of reach until sweet-time. The child knows where they are, when they will be able to eat them and will look forward to this special treat. Encourage the child/parent/guardian not to 'snack' in-between meals. Offer practical suggestions for packed lunches, drinks and meals. A positive attitude and reinforcement of regular visits/attendance should achieve results! It takes time and patience with the whole family unit.

QUESTIONS

?

Question 4

Write some suggestions for a packed lunch, drinks and meals. Don't forget it may be a one-parent family – do you think this makes a difference?

_____

_____

_____

_____

Toothbrushing

There are some things to remember, including:

- ❍ Tell the child to use a small headed toothbrush.

- ❍ Suggest supervised toothbrushing until ten years of age.

- ❍ Confirm that teeth should be brushed twice a day – after breakfast and before going to bed.

- ❍ Confirm that child should use a fluoride toothpaste.

- ❍ Demonstrate the correct toothbrushing technique.

QUESTIONS

?

Question 4

Ask your dentist what advice they give to the parent/guardian and child about toothbrushing.

_____

_____

_____

Fluoride facts

Some important facts include:

○ Fluoride is a natural mineral found in water.

○ The amount of fluoride found in water varies around the UK. The correct quantity of fluoride in water is 1 part per million. More than this will cause FLUOROSIS (mottling of the teeth). Less than this will have no effect on the teeth.

ADVANTAGES	DISADVANTAGES
Strengthens and hardens the teeth.	Must have correct dosage, otherwise fluorosis can occur.
Available in drops/tablet form.	Must take every day to be effective until second teeth have all erupted.
Occurs naturally in water.	Amount varies.
Added to some water supplies.	
Available on prescription at dentist's discretion for specific target groups.	

QUESTIONS

Question 5

a. Write down what the dentist you work with advises about fluoride and why.

_____

_____

b. Find out how much fluoride is in your water supply.

_____

_____

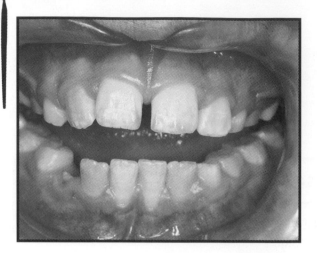

Figure 9.1: Moderate fluorosis caused by ingestion of toothpaste during infancy.

Preparing the child patient for treatment

Actors have a saying 'never work with animals or children'. The idea of dentistry and young children could be seen as equally daunting. The carer will be wondering if their child will 'behave' and not embarrass them. They may themselves be reliving unpleasant dental memories they have experienced and be anxious for their child. The child may not understand what is going to happen or what is expected of them and the dentist may possibly have their own private worries! As dental nurses we can be a bridge between all concerned. We can be the neutral, reassuring and organised link who can respond effectively to all the needs of the participants. This is a vital skill that should not be overlooked and taken for granted.

The child should be told why they are there, what is planned for the visit and shown the equipment that is going to be used and why. It is important that the explanations are given in language that is relevant and meaningful to their age and dental experience. Hiding things and deceiving the child will break the developing bond of trust and prove difficult to re-establish. If something is going to be uncomfortable it is important to say so in a constructive manner.

Giving the child a time frame they can relate to is also advisable. Telling the child that by the count of three it will be done will give them a sense of control and assist in gaining their co-operation for that time period. They also learn to trust the dentist who gives them clearly defined instructions and who does not betray their trust. Effective communication is of paramount importance to successfully treating and developing the child's confidence.

QUESTIONS

Question 6

How does your dental team approach the child patient?

_____

_____

_____

_____

_____

Communication

Effective communication is essential to illustrate how the perception of what is happening can differ. Here are some actual experiences:

What is the problem?

○ The dentist tells an eleven-year-old they are going to take a study model.

○ The child has not experienced this procedure before.

○ The loaded impression tray is put in the child's mouth and starts to set.

○ The child cries profusely.

○ A child of five years has had a glass ionomer restoration placed.

○ They have co-operated throughout and are minutes away from leaving, after a successful visit.

○ The dental nurse is asked for varnish to coat the filling material.

○ With the varnish ready to be placed, the child bursts into tears and is struggling to leave the chair.

With the examples above, there could be a variety of reasons for the problems. Perhaps the dentist did not explain the procedure to the child. The child did not realise the tray contained a material that would set and then the tray would be removed. From the child's point of view this was a form of dental treatment, and the tray would remain in their mouth. This may seem ridiculous to the dental team, who see this type of procedure day in, day out. But is it ridiculous to the child?

Varnish has a strong odour and the child was not warned. They do not know the smell will fade or why it was used. The outcome is that the successful visit became a negative experience, which the child took away with them. The child had behaved well during their first visit for a restoration but it can be easy to become complacent and expect the child to accept everything. Each step must be explained, whether they appear anxious or not.

Common paediatric procedures in primary molars

INDICATIONS FOR	CONTRA-INDICATIONS
Compliance of the child	Uncooperative child
Medical history.	Commitment from parent/guardian
No permanent successor	Medical risks, e.g, bacteria
Masticatory function	More than one tooth involved
Aesthetics	Gross caries (unrestorable tooth)
	Imminent exfoliation

Pulp capping

This procedure is carried out when a pinpoint exposure occurs during cavity preparation. After the decay has been removed and the tooth prepared for the filling material of choice, calcium hydroxide is placed directly on the pinpoint exposure (direct pulp capping) or on a thin residual layer of slightly soft dentine (indirect pulp capping). Calcium hydroxide promotes secondary dentine. The tooth is then lined and amalgam or glass Ionomer is placed.

A pulpotomy is the partial removal of the PULP.

Vital pulpotomies

This procedure involves the removal of the coronal pulp of a vital deciduous molar tooth, which is the name given to the pulp in the crown of the tooth. This may need to be carried out because pulpal exposure more than a pinpoint has occurred during cavity preparation. Invasive caries may also be a cause for considering a vital pulpotomy as the treatment of choice. The aim of the treatment is to maintain the vitality of the radicular pulp. The procedure can be carried out in one visit.

Indications

○ No history/episodes of spontaneous pain.

○ No clinical/radiological evidence of infection.

○ Exposure more than a pinpoint.

○ Carious dentine.

○ Profuse bleeding.

Procedure

○ Administer local anaesthetic.

○ Place rubber dam.

○ Access the tooth using air rotor hand piece and friction grip bur.

○ Remove the coronal pulp with a contra-angled handpiece and rose head bur or a large excavator.

○ Wash and dry the pulp chamber. Use either sterile saline or sterile water in a disposable syringe.

○ Dry the tooth with cotton wool pledgets.

○ Apply formocresol. Dip a sterile pledget into a solution of formocresol and glycerine/glycerol, which should be presented in a glass dappens pot. (Ratio for mixing the two items is: 1 drop formocresol to 4 drops of glycerol). The cotton pledget is left in the pulp chamber for five minutes. This is a hazardous material and should be handled and dispensed with care.

○ Remove the pledget after five minutes. If bleeding has stopped, the tooth can be filled with zinc oxide/eugenol. If residual bleeding continues, repeat the process. A stainless steel crown is usually placed following this procedure to strengthen the roots, which are thin and splayed. This can be done at the same appointment or at a further date.

Non-vital pulpotomies

A non-vital pulpotomy is carried out on a tooth that has had a history of pain and infection. The aim of the procedure is to maintain the structure of the tooth. The coronal pulp is removed and the radicular pulp is treated by a disinfection process using beechwood creosote. The procedure requires two appointments.

Indications

- History/episodes of spontaneous pain.
- Swelling, redness, pain of mucosa.
- Sinus present.
- Tooth mobility.
- Tender to percussion.
- Radiological evidence, e.g, pathological root resorption, bone loss, tooth does not bleed.

First appointment

- Place rubber dam.
- Prepare cavity with air rotor and friction grip burs.
- Excavate deep caries.
- Remove the roof of the pulp chamber.
- Remove the coronal pulp with a large excavator or contra-angled hand piece with rose head bur.
- Wash and dry the pulp chamber. Use either saline or sterile water in a disposable syringe.
- Dry with sterile cotton pledgets.
- Apply the disinfection material, beechwood creosote. Dip the cotton wool pledget in the solution, which should be presented in a glass dappens pot.
- The cotton wool pledget is placed in the coronal chamber and is sealed in with a temporary dressing of zinc oxide/eugenol. This is left in place for a week to ten days allowing, the disinfection process to occur.

Second appointment

- Remove the temporary dressing.
- Check for signs and symptoms of persistent infection. The process may be carried out a second time if indicated.
- To complete the treatment fill the tooth with zinc oxide and eugenol cement.
- Fit a stainless steel crown.

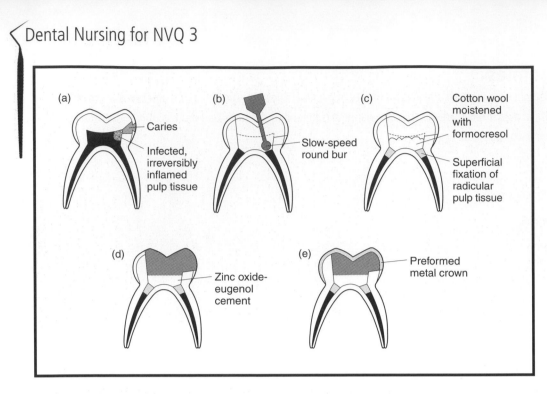

Figure 9.2: Vital pulpotomy

QUESTIONS

?

Question 7

Complete the charts

PULP CAPPING   AIM: _____

                    FEATURE: _____

                    DRESSING: _____

VITAL PULPOTOMY   AIM: _____

                    FEATURE: _____

                    DRESSING: _____

NON-VITAL PULPOTOMY AIM: _____

                    FEATURE: _____

                    DRESSING: _____

QUESTIONS

?

Question 8

What medication do you use in your workplace for vital and non-vital pulpotomies in deciduous molars?

_____

_____

_____

_____

Stainless steel crowns

Stainless steel crowns are also known as preformed metal crowns and were introduced in 1950. Published studies show that stainless steel crowns have a higher success rate in primary teeth than all other restorative materials. They are the preferred treatment option for first primary molars with anything other than minimal caries.

Advantages for stainless steel crowns include the facts that they are:

O   temporary

O   cost effective

O   easy to prepare

O   fast, so require minimal chairtime

O   pliable.

INDICATIONS FOR	CONTRA-INDICATIONS
Compliance	Uncooperative child
Class II cavities	Gross caries (unrestorable tooth)
Enamel defects	Imminent exfoliation
Following a pulpotomy	Aesthetics
Mastication	

Procedure

○ Place bib and safety glasses on the patient.

○ Topical anaesthetic is applied with a cotton wool roll, then local anaesthetic is given.

○ Rubber dam is applied.

○ The cavity is prepared, then, using the air rotor handpiece and a tapered diamond bur, the tooth is prepared for the crown.

○ The dentist then chooses the correct size stainless steel crown and tries it on the tooth; the dentist may need to adjust the stainless steel crown with the contouring pliers and cut to size using bee-bee scissors.

○ A lining material (e.g. calcium hydroxide) is applied inside the tooth, then a restorative material is placed in the cavity (e.g. glass ionomer).

○ Luting glass ionomer is mixed with water on a mixing pad and placed inside the stainless steel crown with a flat plastic.

○ The stainless steel crown is placed over the tooth and the child is asked to bite hard on a cotton wool roll to ensure the crown is fitted correctly. You should hear a popping noise if fitted correctly.

○ The excess cement is removed with a probe or excavator.

○ The rubber dam is removed.

QUESTIONS

?

Question 9

What other uses are there for stainless steel crowns? Ask your dentist!

_____

_____

_____

_____

Traumatised incisors

The definition of trauma is:

○ emotional shock

○ injury

○ wound.

Classification of injury to anterior teeth

- Enamel only or very little dentine involved.
- Enamel and considerable dentine involved, but not involving the pulp.
- Extensive fracture exposing pulp.
- Traumatised tooth that has become non-vital with or without loss of crown structure.
- Teeth loss as a result of trauma.
- Fracture of root with or without crown structure.
- Displacement of tooth with or without fracture of crown or root.
- Fracture of entire crown.

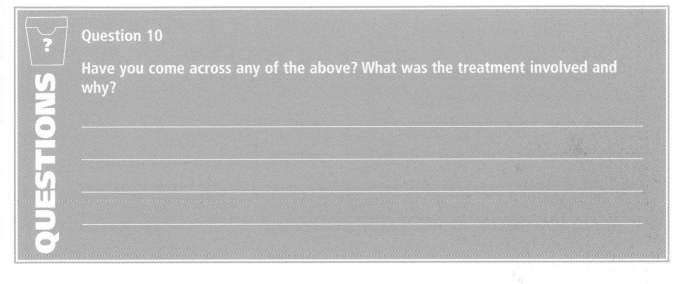

QUESTIONS

?

Question 10

Have you come across any of the above? What was the treatment involved and why?

If the parent/guardian is not happy about the treatment due to the length of procedure/time factor, other options may be considered including:

- the tooth is extracted and a partial denture fitted
- an adhesive retained bridge may be considered when all the permanent teeth have erupted.

☞ Following any episode of trauma to the tooth, there is always a risk of pulpal death as a result. This can occur soon after the accident or up to several years' time. It is important to review clinically and radiographically at regular intervals. The parents and the patient should be warned that any discomfort or discolouring should be reported immediately.

QUESTIONS

Question 11

Ask your dentist about adhesive retained bridges.

_____

_____

_____

_____

_____

Mouth guards

Mouth guards help protect the teeth against trauma. Indications for this include:

○ previous trauma to tooth and continuing treatment.

○ to protect protruding anteriors for those awaiting orthodontic treatment.

○ contact sports – including playing at home with siblings.

Two appointments are required.

First appointment

○ The dentist will select the appropriate size of impression tray, usually an upper and lower impression is required. Fit tray handles. Tray adhesive is applied to the tray.

○ Prepare 2–2 ratio of alginate and water measure. Water at room temperature (21°C) is best. Hot water will make the mix set too quickly and too cold will delay the process causing additional discomfort for the patient.

○ Load impression tray with alginate and hand to the dentist.

○ Keep a kidney dish handy as the procedure can cause the patient to retch.

○ Once both impressions are complete wash under water and place in a disinfectant solution for the required time. Wrap impressions in a damp gauze napkin and place in plastic bag. Make sure laboratory documentation is filled out and all items are identified with patient's details.

○ Give patient mirror and tissues and help patient clean face.

○ Check that the next appointment is made and that laboratory work will be completed by the date given.

Alginate impressions must not be left in the surgery overnight. Alginate impressions will deteriorate and will shrink away from the tray. The work made from this impression will therefore be a distortion of the actual impression and items made from this will not fit. They must be taken to the laboratory so they can be cast.

Second appointment

Always check at the beginning of a treatment session that any laboratory work needed has been returned. If it has not and cannot be delivered before the patient's appointment time, you must cancel the appointment as soon as possible. It is important to arrange a further appointment.

○ The mouth guard will be tried in for fit and comfort.

Care

○ Clean after use.

○ When not in use, store in water in the box provided.

○ Take the mouth guard to each subsequent dental appointment to check for fit/comfort.

Splints

○ Quick and easy to construct.

○ Comfortable.

○ Durable – the splint needs to be in situ for the required length of time to help enable the healing processes to occur.

○ Relatively easy to remove when required.

○ Passive – the splint should not inhibit general function of the mouth as a whole.

Chairside splint

For displaced or avulsed permanent Incisors.

Composite method

○ Place protective glasses and bib on patient.

○ Anaesthetic can be administered if procedure includes repositioning displaced teeth.

○ Use the saliva ejector and cotton wool rolls to increase visibility and keep the area as dry as possible.

○ Apply gel etchant to the teeth that will support the splint and also the teeth that are mobile. Leave for 30 seconds and rinse with the 3-in-1 and dry with the air syringe.

○ Apply bonding agent with disposable brush and light cure.

○ The splint will be attached to all the anterior teeth to form an arch.

○ Cut a piece of 7 mm orthodontic wire to span the number of teeth that are to be splinted. Bend ends of wire round with Adam's pliers so there are no sharp edges.

○ Hold arch wire in position and place composite over wire on each labial surface to be included in the supportive arch.

○ Light cure the composite material for approximately 40 seconds on each tooth. Additional composite may be required to stabilise arch wire. Repeat as required.

Trim method

○ Place protective glasses and bib on patient.

○ Anaesthetic can be administered if procedure includes repositioning displaced teeth.

○ Use the saliva ejector and cotton wool rolls to increase visibility and keep the area as dry as possible.

○ Bend and cut the wire to fit the mobile tooth and two or three adjacent teeth. Bend the cut ends to lie in the embrasures.

○ Wash with air water jet.

○ Isolate the teeth with cotton rolls and dry with air jet.

○ Apply the etching gel to the middle of the labial surfaces with a disposable brush and leave for one minute.

○ Wash away gel for ten seconds, using an aspirator and 3-in-1 syringe.

○ Re-isolate and dry the teeth thoroughly.

○ To apply composite 'trim' use incremental brush technique as follows:

  – liquid in one dappens pot and powder in the other

  – dip the brush in the liquid and then in the powder and carry the resulting mixture to the tooth surface

  – build up 'buttons' of trim on each tooth and then set the wire into the buttons as the material begins to set

  – add further increments to enclose the wire.

☞ Displaced mobile teeth that are to be repositioned should be supported with a finger during the application of the splint.

Laboratory splint

Laboratory splints are made of soft acrylic and look like a mouth guard. They are occasionally used, but accidental avulsion of a previously luxated tooth in the impression material can occur. Laboratory splints compromise oral hygiene and can slow down the healing process of the surrounding tissues.

○ Place bib and safety glasses on the patient.

○ Topical anaesthetic is applied to the area where the trauma has occurred, with a cotton wool roll.

○ Local anaesthetic is given.

○ Teeth are repositioned.

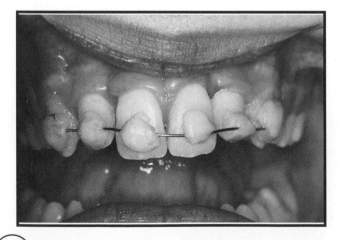

Figure 9.3: Chairside splint.

○ Select impression trays, fit tray handle and apply adhesive.

○ Shake (or fluff) the alginate powder to loosen it, set out a 2–2 ratio of alginate powder and water ready to mix; the water should be neither too hot nor too cold, as this will affect the setting time.

○ Apply a generous amount of Vaseline to the area.

○ When the dentist and patient are ready, start to mix the water and alginate powder together into a smooth consistency.

○ Load the impression tray with the mixture and hand to the dentist.

○ Keep a kidney dish to one side in case the patient has gag reflex.

○ Help the patient clean any debris off their face.

○ Wash the impression under running water and remove tray handle.

○ Place the impression in disinfectant for the required time.

○ Wrap the impression in wet gauze and place in plastic bag, attach the laboratory card.

○ Give the patient a hand mirror to check their appearance.

○ Take the work to the laboratory for the splint to be made.

○ Once splint has been made, fit the splint.

○ Tell the patient how and when to wear it and how to clean it.

○ Give the patient clear oral hygiene instructions.

○ Make another appointment in 7–10 days to review the patient.

☞ Splint remains on for 1–4 weeks, depending on severity of injury, but no longer than a month for root fracture or displacement.

Composite build up

Occurs when the enamel and dentine has fractured on a permanent incisor. The procedure is as follows:

○ Put glasses and bib on patient.

○ Administer local anaesthetic if required.

○ Apply dry dam.

○ Remove any old composite material, if necessary, with an air rotor and FG diamond/tungsten burs.

○ Measure tooth with the dividers. Match the size against the crown form pattern guide to select the appropriate acetate crown form. Cut to size using the Bee-Bee crown scissors.

○ Select the composite shade.

○ Polish the tooth using a bristle brush and contra angle hand piece with pumice mixed with water.

○ Wash and dry.

○ Place gel etchant on the tooth with a disposable brush and leave for 30 seconds.

○ Rinse off with water using the 3-in-1 and suction. Dry the tooth with the 3-in-1 syringe.

○ Apply the bonding agent with a disposable brush, light cure for approximately 20 seconds.

○ Dentist to use probe to pierce corner of mesial edge of crown form to allow air bubbles to be squeezed out.

○ Put the composite into the crown form with a flat plastic 156, a ball ended burnisher may be used to push the material down to eliminate air bubbles.

○ The crown form is then pushed firmly into position onto the remaining part of the existing tooth. Light cure the composite for 40 seconds on both sides. Labial and palatal or lingual and labial.

○ Remove crown form using an excavator or probe.

○ Remove excess composite material with finishing burs and air rotor hand piece.

○ Using polishing and abrasive discs, polish the material starting with a coarse disc and working down through medium, fine and extra fine, to ensure that no ledges or interproximal overhangs are left.

Composite veneers

This method of restoring aesthetics for discoloured teeth in children is useful for the following reasons:

○ The maturing process of the mouth is a gradual one. It is not usually complete until a young person reaches their late teens.

○ Composite veneer is added to the tooth surface and can be replaced in the future if required. It is therefore a non-invasive procedure.

○ As a non-invasive procedure there is no structural removal of tooth required, which, with a view to the future, does not compromise the dental options the patient may choose, e.g, porcelain veneer or porcelain jacket crown.

○ Porcelain veneers or porcelain jacket crowns that are constructed in immature mouths, usually under 16 years old are not desirable. As the mouth matures the gingival margin will change, which creates a gap between the cervical edge of the porcelain and the gum. In addition, the tooth has been structurally altered to accommodate this option and is compromised at an earlier age. Dentistry continues to develop and new materials and options may change in the future. Paediatric care should consider this wherever possible.

The procedure is as follows:

○ Put glasses and bib on patient.

○ Give local anaesthetic if required.

○ Choose shade of composite.

○ Apply dry dam.

○ Polish with pumice.

○ Apply etchant with a disposable brush, leave for 30 seconds, wash off with 3-in-1 syringe and dry.

○ Place bonding agent on tooth with disposable brush and set with light cure; wait for approximately 20 seconds.

○ Using a flat plastic put the composite over the whole surface of the tooth, then light cure. Cure for at least 40 seconds using acetate crown form or layer technique.

○ Remove any unwanted composite with air rotor handpiece and finishing burs.

○ Use discs to smooth and polish the composite, to ensure that the following are checked: gingival margin, interproximal areas and surface ledges.

Root canal treatment (open apex)

The aim of this treatment is to form a dentine bridge to enable the tooth to be root filled.

In immature teeth with an open apex the calcium hydroxide dressing will encourage the formation of a calcified barrier or bridge. This is a natural process requiring time and patience – each individual will be different. It is important that a regular timetable of appointments is kept in order to monitor developments and re-dress the tooth. In general, the following plan would be made.

First appointment

Calcium hydroxide

○ Place bib and safety glasses on the patient.

○ Place rubber dam.

○ Make an access cavity in the palatal or lingual surface of the tooth, using air rotor handpiece and diamond bur.

○ Remove the non-vital pulp tissue, using a barbed broach.

○ Irrigate the canal with sterile water or sodium hypochlorite.

○ Dry the canal using paper points.

○ Fill the canal with non-setting calcium hydroxide, using a contra angle handpiece and spiral root filler or syringe and blunt needle.

○ Place cotton wool pledget at the opening of the tooth.

○ Seal cavity with zinc oxide/eugenol.

○ Remove rubber dam.

○ Take periapical radiograph, if required.

○ Give the patient another appointment to re-dress the tooth. Warn the patient, if the dressing is lost, to contact for earlier appointment.

Following the extirpation procedure and initial placement of calcium hydroxide dressing, the patient would be seen in approximately three weeks to assess and re-dress the tooth. Further visits for replacement dressing would be roughly four to six months apart.

Subsequent appointments

Calcium hydroxide change

○ Place bib and safety glasses on the patient.

○ Place rubber dam, if required.

○ Open the access cavity (palatal or lingual) using air rotor handpiece and diamond bur.

○ Remove cotton wool pledget.

○ Check apical calcific barrier, using small file or paper point.

○ Irrigate the canal with sterile water or sodium hypochlorite.

○ Use file to measure working length of the canal.

○ Take periapical radiograph.

○ Irrigate the canal again.

○ Dry the canal using paper points.

○ Fill the canal with non-setting calcium hydroxide, using a contra angle handpiece and spiral root filler or syringe and blunt needle.

○ Place cotton wool pledget at the opening of the tooth.

○ Seal cavity using zinc oxide/eugenol.

○ Remove rubber dam.

○ Take another periapical radiograph, if required.

○ Give the patient another appointment, to re-dress the tooth. Warn the patient, if the dressing is lost, to contact for earlier appointment.

☞ This would continue until radiographic and clinical examination provided evidence that the barrier had developed. The next stage would be to arrange obturation of the canal, which means it would be filled with a permanent material. Replacement of calcium hydroxide is carried out for up to two years, after which time the treatment plan is reviewed.

QUESTIONS

Question 11

Find out why the permanent material is not placed until the barrier has formed.

_____

_____

_____

_____

_____

☞ It would be advisable to postpone the obturation stage if orthodontic work is planned. It is considered less stressful for the tooth during orthodontic movement if it contains a dressing, rather than a rigid filling material that is not flexible.

Question 12

a Can you give reasons for this?

_____

_____

b. Ask your dentist to show you radiographs demonstrating open and closed apex.

_____

_____

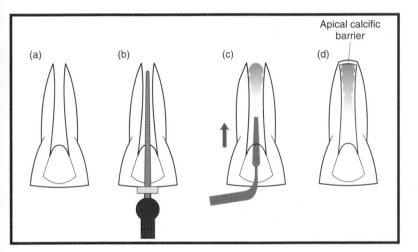

Figure 9.4: Diagram of an open apex.

Internal bleaching non-vital teeth 'walking bleach'

When considering methods to reduce or remove tooth discolouration, internal bleaching is a non-invasive technique that is only suitable for non-vital teeth.

This procedure utilises the root filled pulp chamber of the tooth. Discolouration of the tooth following pulp death creates a degree of shadow, which is visible. By placing the bleaching agent inside the tooth for a set period of time, the degree of staining can be reduced with varying degrees of success. The extent of discolouration is a factor and the level of acceptance of the appearance by the patient. Each case is different and the changes in colour will vary. Generally, no more than three visits to assess the changes and replace the material would complete this option. Before considering other procedures, which involve treating the external surface, this is a useful first step to attempt.

- Place safety glasses and plastic bib on the patient.

- Ensure both sinks are filled with cold water, for the instruments and items to be placed in when finished with.

- Clean teeth with pumice using contra-angle hand piece, prophy head and bristle brush.

- Make note of the shade of the discoloured tooth.

- Apply rubber dam, isolating the tooth.

- Remove palatal restoration and pulp chamber restoration using an air rotor hand piece and bur.

- Ensure that the root filling completely seals the canal to prevent any of the chemicals permeating the root canal.

- Place a lining of zinc phosphate cement into the base of the pulp chamber to cover the root filling.

- Sodium perborate crystals moistened with sterile water in a glass dappens pot.

- Sodium perborate crystals are placed into the root canal using a large excavator.

- Cotton wool pledgets are then placed in the canal before sealing the access cavity with zinc oxide/eugenol.

- Remove rubber dam.

- Review the patient in 7–10 days to assess colouration changes. Repeat the procedure if necessary. No more than three visits are usually needed depending on the progress made each time. If the procedure has proved unsatisfactory other options will have to be considered.

Health and safety

- Keep bleaching materials on the clinician's side.

- Fill sinks with cold water to dilute bleaching agent.

- Always use a plastic bib.

- Do not pass things over the face.

- Rinse well before removing rubber dam.

Introduction

This chapter is linked to DN24 of the NVQ Level 3 in Oral Health Care.

Orthodontics could be defined as that area of dentistry specialising in the study of growth and development of the teeth and facial skeleton, and the treatment of irregularities of the teeth and jaws.

A qualified and registered dentist may carry out orthodontic treatment. A dentist who has undertaken a recognised course of further training in orthodontics can apply to be placed on the specialist orthodontic list held by the General Dental Council (GDC). Orthodontists may work in a dental practice, within an outpatients' department of a hospital, a dental teaching institute or community clinic.

SECTION 1:   Anatomy and physiology

Before looking more closely at the treatment side of orthodontics it is important that some basic understanding of anatomy and physiology involving the teeth and jaws is established. Subject areas to be covered are:

- The tooth and its supporting structures

- Specific features of the teeth

- The muscles of mastication

- Deciduous and permanent eruption dates

- The relationship of the upper and lower jaws

- Occlusion and malocclusion

- The process of tooth movement.

The tooth and its supporting structures

The tooth comprises the crown, which is visible in the oral cavity and the root, which is embedded within the bone of the jaws, and is not normally visible in health. The main parts of a tooth are the enamel, dentine and pulp (Figure 10.1). The tooth is supported within the alveolar bone of the upper maxilla and lower mandible by ligaments and a cement-like substance covering the root called cementum. The alveolar bone is covered by a tissue known as the gingiva, which also acts as a support structure to the tooth. Each tooth has certain features that will make it possible to distinguish it from another tooth. In orthodontics some of these features are used to measure irregularities in the way teeth fit together and also to measure tooth movement and determine completion of treatment.

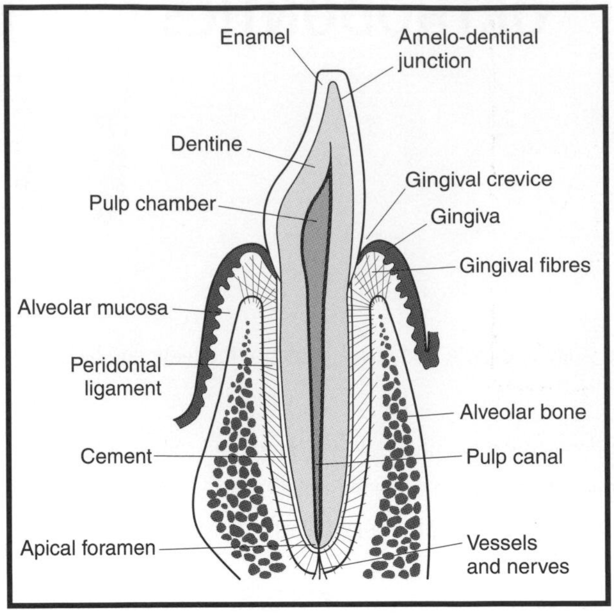

Figure 10.1: Cross section of a single-rooted tooth.

Specific features of the teeth

The surfaces of the crowns of the teeth are given specific names in order to make life easier and to establish some degree of standardisation when describing an area of a tooth. Below is a list of specific features and where they may be located on a tooth (see Figures 10.2 and 10.3).

○ Proximal surfaces – Each tooth has two proximal surfaces. The surface nearest the mid-line of the face is the mesial proximal surface and the surface furthest away from the mid-line of the face is the distal proximal surface.

○ Buccal – that part of the tooth that faces the cheek.

○ Labial – that part of the tooth that faces the lips.

○ Lingual – that part of the tooth that faces the tongue.

○ Palatal – that part of the tooth that faces the palate.

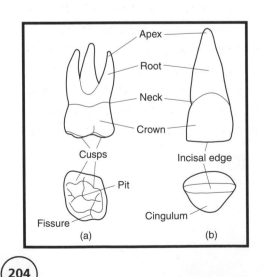

Figure 10.2: Anatomical landmarks in upper molar (a) and upper incisor (b).

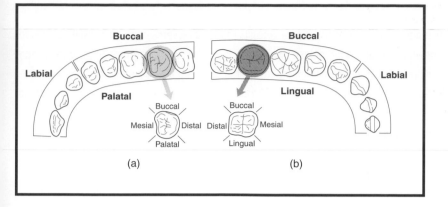

Figure 10.3: Tooth surfaces in the maxila (a) and mandible (b).

❍ Incisal edge/ridge – found on the biting surfaces of incisor and canine teeth.

❍ Occlusal surfaces – located on the biting surfaces of premolars and molars.

❍ Cusps – projections on the occlusal and incisal surfaces of canines, premolars and molars. Incisors do not have cusps.

❍ Cingulum – a rounded projection found lingually and palatally on the incisors and canines. It lies near to the gingival margin and is particularly prominent on the palatal surfaces of the maxillary canines.

❍ Developmental grooves – lines that are left after the tooth has finished developing. They can be seen most clearly on the molars on the buccal surfaces running between the cusps.

Enamel

The outer covering of the crown is made up of a mineral called enamel, which is whitish in colour and is the hardest substance in the body. If viewed under the microscope, millions of interlocking crystals made up of a material similar to a substance known as hydroxyapatite may be seen. These crystals run from the inner to the outer surface of enamel and are known as enamel rods or prisms. Although these crystals are hard they are susceptible to being dissolved by acids such as those produced by bacterial plaque. Enamel does not contain nerves or blood vessels and therefore is insensitive to pain.

Dentine

The next layer of the tooth is made up of a partially mineralised substance known as dentine, which lies under the enamel of the crown and also forms the outer surface of the root. Dentine is yellowish in colour and is also made up of crystals of hydroxyapatite but in smaller concentrations than enamel. Dentine is softer than enamel but harder than bone. When viewed under a microscope thousands of small channels known as dentinal tubules will be seen running from the inner surface of the dentine to the junction with the enamel. These tubules contain cell processes, which come from cells lining the pulp chamber, called odontoblasts. Odontoblasts continue to lay down new dentine throughout the life of the tooth, and they also lay down more dentine in response to a stimulus such as dental caries. This helps to protect the pulp from damage and keep the tooth alive. Unlike enamel, dentine can feel the sensation of pain due to its connection with the pulp.

Pulp

The pulp chamber and canals lie under the dentine and contain a soft tissue that consists of blood vessels, lymphatic vessels and nerves, which keep the tooth alive. As mentioned in the previous section, odontoblasts, which line the pulpal walls, continue to produce dentine throughout life; this has the effect of making the pulp chamber and canals smaller over time. The pulp feels pain and can become infected, which may then lead to pulp death and death of the tooth. The nerves and blood vessels leave the pulp canal via a small hole or foramen located at the apex of the root.

Cementum

Cementum covers the root of the tooth and is yellowish in colour. Approximately half of its structure is mineralised with hydroxyapatite, the other half consisting of an organic material and water. The cementum is an important support structure of the tooth, because it is one half of the attachment for the periodontal ligament that holds the tooth in the alveolar bone.

The periodontal ligament

The periodontal ligament consists of many collagen fibres that generally run from the cementum on the root to the alveolar bone (Figure 10.4). The periodontal ligament also contains blood vessels, lymphatic vessels and nerves. It is interesting to note that the nerves of the pulp can only transmit pain impulses to the brain, whilst those of the periodontal ligament also transmit sensations of light touch and pressure. This is an important issue when carrying out orthodontic treatment, because movement of the tooth affects the periodontal ligament and this can lead to discomfort for the patient. The periodontal ligament also acts as a kind of 'shock absorber' so that when pressure is applied to the tooth, for example when biting down, it allows the tooth to move a fraction in the socket. If a tooth were stuck rigid in alveolar bone it would probably crack under the stress of biting.

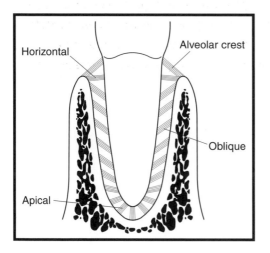

Figure 10.4: Periodontal ligament fibres.

The alveolar bone

The alveolar bone makes up the bone in the socket in the upper jaw (maxilla) and the lower jaw (mandible). Alveolar bone consists of two main layers (see Figure 10.5); compact bone and spongy or cancellous bone. The compact bone is found on the buccal and lingual surfaces of the jaws and also lining the socket. The compact bone of the socket is slightly different from that on the outer surfaces as it consists of many tiny holes, which allow access of blood vessels to the tooth. It is important that bone has a good blood supply because

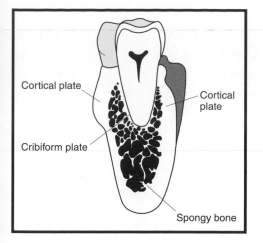

Figure 10.5: Cross section through the mandible showing the layers of alveolar bone.

it is a dynamic structure that is constantly changing and remodelling. ☞ This process of remodelling is important in orthodontic treatment and tooth movement. Bone contains cells called osteoblasts, which lay down new bone, and osteoclasts, which destroy bone. With these two types of cells working together tooth movement without the loss of the tooth is possible.

The gingiva

The gingiva covers the alveolar bone, and forms part of the support structure of the tooth (Figure 10.6). There are two main parts to the gingiva, the marginal gingival (also known as the free gingiva), which forms a cuff about 1–2 mm wide around the neck of the tooth and the attached gingiva, which is connected to the underlying alveolar bone. The marginal gingival can be pulled away from the side of the tooth with a probe as it is not attached to any underlying structure (hence the name free gingiva). The gap between the tooth and the marginal gingiva is known as the gingival sulcus, and in health can be between 0–2 mm in depth. The attached gingiva, when healthy, is pink in colour (with variations for ethnicity) and its surface appear to be stippled. The gingiva between the teeth is known as the interdental papilla.

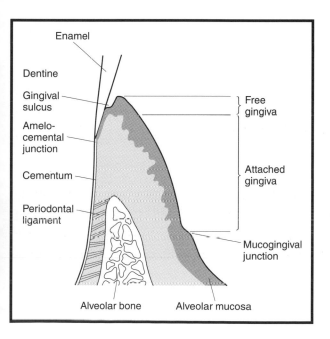

Figure 10.6: Features of the peridontium.

QUESTIONS

? Question 1

Draw and label a diagram of a tooth.

The muscles of mastication

The muscles of mastication are four pairs of muscles attached to the mandible and primarily responsible for:

○ elevating (raising)

○ protruding (pushing out)

○ retruding (pulling back)

○ causing the mandible to move laterally (move to the side).

☞ The muscles of mastication can be utilised when using functional appliances in orthodontic treatment. The mandible is held in a forward position so that wearing the functional appliance uses the action of the muscles. These appliances are most effective when facial growth is still taking place.

RELATED TERMS

Origin – the origin of a muscle is the end of the muscle that is attached to the least moveable structure.

Insertion – the insertion of a muscle is the end of the muscle that is attached to the more moveable structure.

Action – the action is the work that is accomplished when the muscle's fibres contract.

The masseter (Figure 10.7)

Description – a strong quadrilateral muscle.

Origin – originates from the zygomatic arch.

Insertion – the fibres are inserted into the outer surface of the angle of the mandible.

Action – when the muscle contracts, it raises the mandible, closing the mouth.

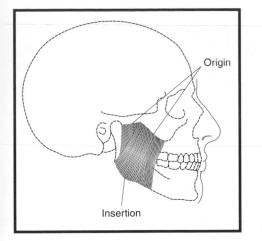

Figure 10.7: Lateral view of the skull showing origin and insertion of masseter muscle.

The temporal – temporalis (Figure 10.8)

Description – a large fan-shaped muscle.

Origin – the temporal bone.

Insertion – the fibres are inserted into the coronoid process and border of the ramus of the mandible.

Action – if the entire muscle contracts the mandible is raised, so closing the mouth. If only part of the muscle contracts it will pull the mandible backward, which is referred to as retruding the mandible.

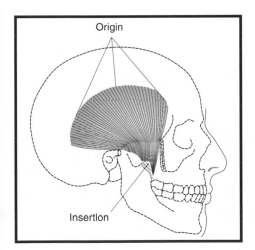

Figure 10.8: Lateral view of the skull showing origin and insertion of temporal muscle.

The medial pterygoid (the 'P' is silent) (Figure 10.9)

Description – a quadrilateral muscle.

Origin this muscle mainly originates from a bone in the skull called the pterygoid plate.

Insertion – it is inserted into the inner surface of the angle of the mandible.

Action – when the muscle contracts, it raises the mandible and closes the mouth.

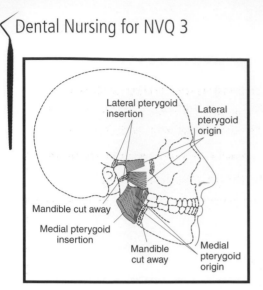

Figure 10.9: Lateral view of the skull showing origin and insertion of medial and lateral Pteygoid muscles.

The lateral pterygoid (Figure 10.9)

Description – triangular shaped muscle.

Origin – from two bones inside the skull, one of which is the pterygoid plate and the other is called the sphenoid bone.

Insertion – inserts into the temporomandibular joint.

Action – helps to protrude and lower the mandible so opening the mouth. Also, when only one of the pair of muscles is working, there will be side movement of the mandible known as lateral excursion to the opposite side of the contracted muscle.

QUESTIONS

?

Question 2

Design a chart giving the name of each muscle with the appropriate origin, insertion and action.

Deciduous and permanent eruption dates

☞ Eruption dates are an important aspect of orthodontic treatment as they help dictate the best time to carry out treatment. There is individual variation concerning the eruption of teeth, however, the tables below show the approximate or average eruption dates for both the deciduous and permanent dentition.

The deciduous dentition (Table 10.1)

There are 20 deciduous teeth, ten in the mandible and ten in the maxilla, with the mandibular teeth generally erupting before those in the maxilla. Root development is normally complete 1–1$^1/_2$ years after tooth eruption and generally all teeth will be erupted by 2$^1/_2$ years. Also note that the sequence of eruption is A B D C E, the canines erupting after the first molars. There are no premolars in the deciduous dentition.

Tooth	Tooth letter	Approximate range of eruption dates
Central incisors	A	6–8 months
Lateral incisors	B	7–9 months
Canines	C	16–20 months
First molars	D	12–15 months
Second molars	E	20–30 months

Table 10.1: Approximate eruption dates for deciduous teeth

There are 32 teeth in the permanent dentition (including the wisdom teeth), 16 in the mandible and 16 in the maxilla, with the mandibular teeth generally erupting before those in the maxilla. Root development is normally complete about three years after tooth eruption.

The permanent dentition (Table 10.2)

Maxillary teeth	Tooth number	Approximate date of eruption
Central incisor	1	7–7$^1/_2$ years
Lateral incisors	2	8–8$^1/_2$ years
Canines	3	11–11$^1/_2$ years
First premolar	4	10 years
Second premolar	5	11 years
First molar	6	6 years
Second molar	7	12 years
Third molar	8	18–25 years
Mandibular teeth		
Central incisor	1	6–6$^1/_2$ years
Lateral incisors	2	7–7$^1/_2$ years
Canines	3	10 years
First premolar	4	10–10$^1/_2$ years
Second premolar	5	11 years
First molar	6	6 years
Second molar	7	12 years
Third molar	8	18–25 years

Table 10.2: Approximate eruption dates for permanent teeth

QUESTIONS

?

Question 3

Learn the eruption dates of the deciduous and permanent dentition.

SECTION 2:   The relationship between the upper and lower jaws

Occlusion and malocclusion

Occlusion may be defined as contact between the occlusal surfaces of the teeth in the upper and lower jaws. In general, the teeth in the maxilla normally overlap those in the mandible, allowing the jaws to fit together in such a way that allows proper function and maintenance of an ideal tooth relationship. However, for a lot of people, that ideal jaw and tooth relationship does not exist, and this may be defined as malocclusion. Malocclusion can include irregularities of individual teeth and/or irregularities in the way that the bones of the skull have developed.

There are a few more definitions that will be useful to know when studying the subject of orthodontics, which are set out in the list below.

○ Overjet – how far *forward* the upper incisors are from the lower incisors

○ Overbite – how far the upper incisors *overlap* the lower incisors

○ Proclined – positioned in front of

○ Retroclined – positioned behind.

Classification of malocclusion

To help orthodontists clarify the many types of malocclusion, a system of classification has been established of which there are two main types. Both types are often used in conjunction with one another.

Angle's classification

A classification system that is universally recognised is Angle's classification, based on the relationship between the upper and lower jaws as measured from front to back (known as the sagittal plane). The important relationship in Angle's classification is how the upper and lower first permanent molars occlude with each other. In an 'ideal relationship' the anterior buccal grove of the lower first permanent molar should occlude with the anterior buccal cusp of the upper first permanent molar (Figure 10.10).

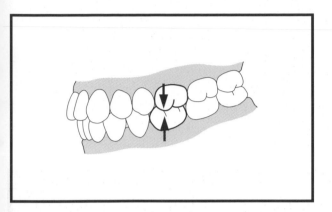

Figure 10.10: Angle's Class 1 occlusal relationship.

Incisor classification (Figure 10.11)

Another classification system uses the relationship between the upper and lower incisors. This classification has often proved to be more useful to orthodontists, as the majority of treatment is carried out for aesthetic purposes.

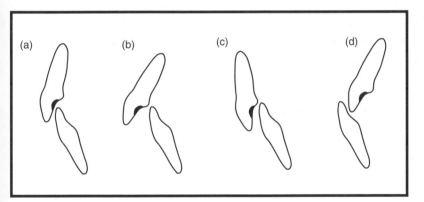

Figure 10.11: Incisor classification.

Incisor relationships

Class I

○ The lower incisor edge occludes with the middle third of the palatal aspect of the upper incisors.

○ Overjet and overbite are normal but there may be crowding, impaction and displacement of teeth.

○ Angle's class I molar relationship.

Class II division 1

○ The lower incisor edges lie posterior to the cingulum of the upper incisors.

○ Upper incisors are proclined.

○ There is an increased overjet and overbite is frequently increased.

○ Angle's class II molar relationship.

Class II division 2

○ Occurs in approximately ten per cent of the population.

○ Increased overbite.

○ Upper central incisors may be retroclined and upper lateral incisors may be proclined.

○ Lower anterior teeth are frequently retroclined.

○ In severe cases lower incisors may occlude with palatal mucosa.

Class III

○ Found in approximately three per cent of the population.

○ The lower incisor tips lie anterior to the palatal cingulum of the upper incisors.

○ Frequently there is a reversed overjet. The lower anterior teeth lie infront of the upper anterior teeth.

○ Upper incisors are often crowded and usually proclined.

○ There may be a deep overbite.

The process of tooth movement

☞ There are two main tooth movements that are useful for a DN to understand, one is tipping and the other is bodily movement and rotation.

Tipping

This is where there is a light force applied to the crown of the tooth leaving the root in the same position. This type of movement is usually achieved using a removable orthodontic appliance (Figure 10.12).

Bodily movement and rotation

This is where two forces are applied causing both the crown and the root to move. A fixed orthodontic appliance would be necessary to achieve this type of movement.

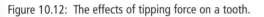

Figure 10.12: The effects of tipping force on a tooth.

Changes in the support structures of the teeth during movement

Changes in the tissues of the support structures of the teeth are dependent on how much force is applied and for how long. About 24 hours after a forced is applied to a tooth the periodontal ligament will undergo tension and compression. In other words, the periodontal ligament is stretched one side and squashed the other as it is being pulled in one direction. With continued force the alveolar bone lining the socket is resorbed by oestoclasts on the side that the tooth is moving toward, and oestoblasts lay down bone behind it. With slow and constant force the tooth can move without the risk of damage to the root surface (root resorption) or the supporting structures such as the periodontal ligament and alveolar bone.

After treatment is complete, there will have to be a period of retention where the teeth are held in a fixed position. This is to allow time for the bone and periodontal ligament to settle down and for the teeth to become firm within the socket.

SECTION 3:   Orthodontic treatment planning linked to DN24.2, DN24.3

The quality of the treatment outcome is very much dependent on careful planning by the orthodontist. The course of orthodontic treatment may take place over an extended period, and is often dependent on the patient's growth and development. In the planning phase of treatment the orthodontist has to predict the end result and literally has to 'see into the future'. Treatment planning will provide a systematic approach to the diagnosis, treatment and care of the patient, so that the best possible results are achieved. This section will look at all the aspects that go into planning orthodontic treatment for a patient.

Topics covered in this section:

○ The aims of orthodontic treatment

○ Orthodontic treatment options

○ Patient selection

○ Timescales of treatment

○ Benefits of treatment

○ The potential risk of orthodontic treatment

○ Diagnostic aids to orthodontic treatment.

Orthodontic treatment aims

Probably the most common aim when carrying out orthodontic treatment is to improve the look (aesthetics) of the face and teeth. However, orthodontic treatment may also aim to deal with the following:

○ improving the function of the teeth

○ moving teeth that may be at risk from trauma

○ moving teeth to eliminate stagnation areas

○ aligning the teeth ready for crown and bridge work

○ aligning teeth to aid oral hygiene

○ placing the teeth and jaws in the correct position for surgery (orthognathic surgery).

Orthodontic treatment options

There are several options available to the orthodontist when planning a patient's treatment. The simplest option is to do nothing and accept the malocclusion if it is mild, and where treatment may not produce any obvious benefits to the patient. Other treatment options include:

○ extracting the teeth to relieve crowding but not fitting any orthodontic appliance

○ using removable appliances

○ using fixed appliances

○ using functional appliances

○ orthographic surgery

○ utilisation of headgear.

All of the above may be used in conjunction with one another. For example, a patient may start with a functional appliance, then have fixed appliances placed and then wear a removable non-active appliance as a retainer. Headgear may be worn with either removable or fixed appliances. Orthognathic surgery involves moving the jaws and is usually only carried out in patients with severe malocclusions and where orthodontic appliances would not fully complete the treatment.

Patient selection for orthodontic treatment

Patients are normally referred by their GDP to either an orthodontic practice, an orthodontic department in a local general hospital, a dental teaching institute or community clinic. Children as well as adults can be referred, although the majority of referrals are for children between the ages of 9 and 12. Before embarking on any orthodontic treatment the following factors need to be considered:

- severity of the malocclusion;

- the age of the patient;

- deciduous, mixed or permanent dentition;

- the medical history of the patient;

- the oral hygiene status of the patient;

- any dental diseases that may be present, such as dental caries or periodontal disease;

- patient motivation for treatment;

- parent motivation for treatment;

- the patient's expectations of treatment;

- the patient's psychological condition;

- if the patient has any special needs;

- cost of treatment if the patient is paying;

- whether the patient would benefit from being treated in a hospital or practice environment.

The timescales of orthodontic treatment

Orthodontic treatment can be lengthy, taking from a few months to a few years. This is why it is so important to try and establish the patient's motivation and commitment to treatment during the treatment planning stage. ☞ The unmotivated or non-compliant patient may disrupt the course of treatment and cause the outcome to be compromised, possibly resulting in long-term dental health problems. Once treatment has commenced patients usually attend for an appointment about every four to six weeks.

The benefits of orthodontic treatment

The most obvious benefit to the patient is an improvement in facial and dental aesthetics. This may have a psychological effect and increase the patient's confidence both in a professional and social context. With severe malocclusions, function will be improved and trauma to dental tissues reduced or eliminated.

The potential risks of orthodontic treatment

As with any treatment there will always be potential risks involved, and orthodontic treatment is no exception. During treatment planning the orthodontist would decide if the potential risks to the patient outweigh the benefits of treatment. These are only potential risks, and often a lot will depend not only on the expertise of the orthodontist, but also the compliance of the patient during treatment. Potential risks may include:

○ demineralisation of tooth structure leading to white spot lesions and dental caries;

○ periodontal disease;

○ trauma from intra oral appliances;

○ trauma from headgear;

○ allergies to appliances;

○ root resorption;

○ death of the pulp;

○ residual spacing after treatment.

👉 Other risk factors that need to be taken into consideration include protection of the patient during clinical procedures, radiation protection, and infection control procedures.

Diagnostic aids to orthodontic treatment

Before orthodontic treatment can begin certain measurements need to be taken to help formulate a diagnosis (what the problem is) and treatment plan (how best to deal with the problem). These measurements are normally taken at the initial visit and may include:

○ radiographs;

○ impressions for study models;

○ photographs.

Radiographs

Radiographs provide a method by which a detailed analysis of facial structures can be carried out, as well as providing an overview of the position of erupted and unerupted teeth. Radiographs that are normally taken for orthodontic diagnosis include:

○ Lateral cephalometric (Figure 10.13) – this shows a side view of the skull, upper and lower jaws and the relationship between hard and soft tissues. This radiograph is used in conjunction with the clinical findings, as a diagnostic aid. The use of two or more views over a period of time can assess the growth of the developing face and dentition.

○ Orthopantomogram (Figure 10.14) – used to show the development of all the teeth, erupted and unerupted, the maxillary sinuses and the temporomandibular joints features such as alveolar bone levels, supernumerary teeth, restorations present and pathology of the jaws.

○ Upper central/anterior occlusal views (Figure 10.15) – can be used to locate supernumerary teeth. This figure also shows the upper incisor teeth, their supporting bone and the anterior part of the palate.

Study models

Study models are used to evaluate the occlusion, diagnose malocclusion and record changes due to natural development or treatment. A wax bite is normally taken at the same time to record the patient's normal occlusion when they bite together. This will aid the dental technician in ensuring the correct relationship of the casts (Figure 10.16).

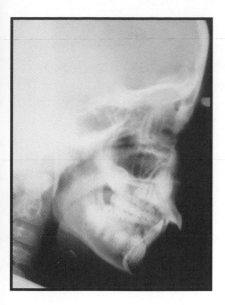

Figure 10.13: Lateral cephalometric skull.

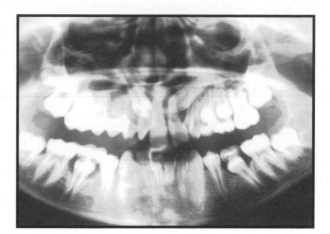

Figure 10.14: An orthopantomograph.

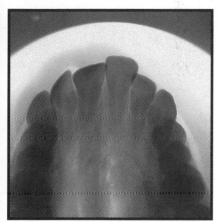

Figure 10.15: An upper anterior occlusal radiograph.

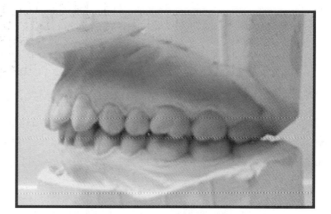

Figure 10.16: Study models

Photographs

Intra oral and extra oral photographs will help to record the dental health and the facial features of the patient prior to treatment. Before and after photographs can often be a motivating factor for the patient, and also useful as a teaching resource. Patients need to give their consent for their photographs to be used for teaching purposes.

Types of appliance and their components

As described in the section on treatment options, there are numerous different types of orthodontic appliance and each one has a specific action. The appliances that will be described include:

○ removable appliances

○ functional appliances

○ fixed appliances.

The use of headgear will also be covered in this section.

Removable appliances

☞ These appliances can be taken out of the mouth during treatment by the patient for cleaning purposes only. On occasions they may be removed when playing a contact sport. Removable appliances may either be active (moving teeth) or passive (holding teeth in a certain position).

Removable appliances – components and use (Figure 10.17)

○ Acrylic baseplate – retains the appliance in the mouth and provides attachment for the active and retentive components of the appliance

○ Retention – includes Adams cribs

○ Active components – includes springs, labial bows, and screws.

☞ An alginate impression and wax bite is taken of the patient's mouth, and from this the removable appliance is constructed in the laboratory by a technician. As well as a written description of the appliance, the orthodontist provides a detailed diagram for the technician to ensure accuracy. Removable appliances may be used for:

○ tipping the teeth (the root will stay in its original position)

○ rotating the teeth (if rotation is mild)

○ reducing some overbites

○ maintaining space between teeth

○ holding the teeth in position after fixed appliance treatment, (known as retention).

Removable appliances cannot move the roots of the teeth through bone and are therefore usually only used for simple malocclusions, or in conjunction with fixed appliances. ☞ It is important that the patient wears them as instructed by the orthodontist or treatment will not be successful. Removable appliances may be damaged if they are not worn as prescribed, so the patent should be advised to remove them only for cleaning or some contact sports. If the appliance is removed from the mouth it should be kept in a rigid plastic

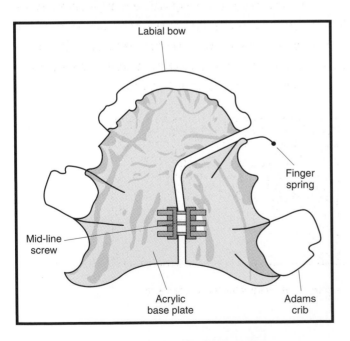

Figure 10.17: An upper removable orthodontic appliance.

lidded container for protection. If the appliance does become broken it should be returned to the orthodontist as soon as possible for repair. When the appliance is out of the mouth for even a short period of time the teeth may begin to return to their original position, resulting in the appliance not fitting properly and delaying treatment. ☞ The dental nurse may be given the role of informing the patient on how to fit and remove their orthodontic appliance safely and also on appliance care. The patient attends for an orthodontic appointment every four to six weeks to have the appliance checked and adjusted.

Functional appliances

As mentioned in section one, functional appliances utilise the action of the muscles of mastication to effect tooth movement. Functional appliances are most effective when the patient is going though a period of rapid growth, which is normally during puberty. Functional appliance therapy can be followed by removable or fixed appliance treatment.

Functional appliances – components and use

☞ An alginate impression and wax bite is taken and the technician, following the orthodontist's description and design, constructs the functional appliance. There are several different types of functional appliance but only three will be mentioned here.

The Andresen appliance – consists largely of one block of acrylic that fits both the maxilla and mandible and is held in place by a labial bow. Modern activating appliances based on the Andresen design may be known as bionators, (figure 10.18). It opens the bite and encourages the mandible to be held in a forward position. This type of functional appliance can be used for patients with Class II Division 1 malocclusions. ☞ It should be worn every night and as much as possible during the day. The appliance has to be taken out for eating and contact sports. Speech will be affected to begin with but the patient will adapt when they get used to wearing it.

The Frankel appliance (Figure 10.19) – This functional appliance consists of 'pads' of acrylic that hold the lips and cheeks away from the teeth. It affects both the position of the mandible and the contour of the facial soft tissues and is most commonly used to treat Class II Division 1 malocclusions. A mesh of carefully constructed wires holds the pads of acrylic together. This appliance can be bulky and uncomfortable for the patent to wear initially and will affect speech to some degree. The appliance is taken out for eating and contact sports.

The twin block appliance (Figure 10.20) – This functional appliance consists of two separate upper and lower acrylic plates that are retained by Adams cribs. On each plate are posterior bite blocks, which encourage the patient to push the mandible forward in order to achieve a comfortable position. ☞ This appliance is used to treat moderate to severe Class II Division 1 malocclusions. As the appliance is not fused together it can be more comfortable for the patient to wear than the other functional appliances, and has less effect on speech. It can be worn practically full-time and is usually only removed for cleaning and contact sports.

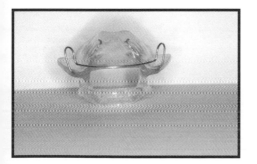

Figure 10.18: Bionator activator appliance (modern form of Andresen appliance).

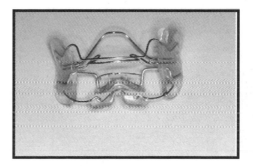

Figure 10.19: Frankel functional appliance.

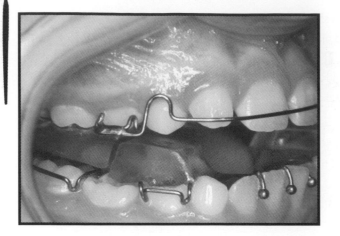

Figure 10.20: Twin block appliance.

Fixed appliances

Fixed appliances are not constructed outside the mouth by a technician, but consist of brackets, bands and wires that are attached to the teeth whilst in the dental chair. Fixed appliances move the root through bone so, unlike removable appliances, the whole tooth moves rather than just the crown being tipped. The action of fixed appliances allows the orthodontist more scope to treat severe malocclusions.

Fixed appliances – components and uses

The main components of a fixed appliance include (Figure 10.21):

○ **Brackets** – bonded directly to the patient's teeth using either acid etched composites or glass ionomer cements. Brackets include a slot for the arch wire to sit in. Hooks may be attached to the brackets to allow placement of intra oral elastics.

○ **Bands** – normally cemented to the molar teeth using glass ionomer cements. These are rings of metal to fit molars and premolars. Molar bands have buccal tubes for placement of the arch wire.

○ **Wires** – the arch wire slots into the grooves in the brackets and the tubes in the bands to bring about tooth movement.

○ **Elastic modules** – attach the wires to the brackets.

○ **Wire ligatures** – also attach the wire to the brackets.

There are several types of fixed appliance, but only one will be mentioned here.

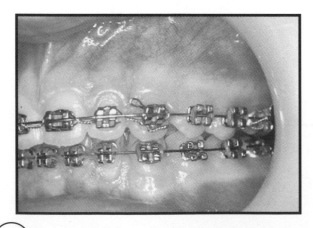

Figure 10.21: A fixed appliance showing brackets, bands, archwire, ligatures and elastic modules.

The 'straight wire' appliance

One of the most popular types of fixed appliance is known as the 'straight wire' appliance. The important aspect of this appliance is the way that each bracket has been designed specifically for individual teeth. Each bracket varies slightly in thickness to compensate for the different thickness of each tooth. The slot on each bracket also matches the inclination (torque), and angulation (tip), of each tooth. Pressure or force is placed on the crown of the tooth by the wire trying to straighten itself whist in the slot of the bracket.

☞ A series of arch wires are placed during the treatment. In the initial stages these apply light aligning forces and are usually made of a thin and very flexible nickel titanium alloy (Ni Ti) wire. As treatment progresses, thicker wire of rectangular cross section is used and may be stainless steel or nickel titanium alloy.

Fixed appliances can be used in conjunction with removable appliances, functional appliances and in preparation for orthognathic surgery.

Headgear (Figure 10.22)

Headgear may be used in conjunction with removable, functional or fixed appliance therapy. It may consist of the following components:

- ⭘ neck strap
- ⭘ head strap
- ⭘ face bow
- ⭘ extra oral elastics or modules.

The headgear may be attached to an appliance either by the ends of the face bow slotting into the buccal tubes on molars bands, or by 'J' hooks attached to labial bows or archwires. Headgear may be used for anchorage to hold the teeth in one position whilst others are being moved, or for movement of the teeth. The force applied by headgear is usually for distal movement of the molar teeth.

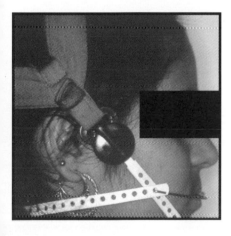

Figure 10.22: Headgear.

SECTION 4: Clinical stages and the role of the DN during orthodontic treatment

☞ The clinical stages and role of the DN may differ from one orthodontic clinic to another depending on such variables as treatment availability, laboratory services and staff resources. Outlined below is a generalisation of what might take place over a number of visits for both removable and fixed appliance treatments.

First visit

Preparation of clinical area

☞ All non-metal surfaces should be disinfected with a solution such as hypochlorite 1.0%. Zone your clinical area into dirty and clean areas and remove any unnecessary items from work surfaces. During this procedure the DN must be wearing protective equipment such as gloves, glasses and mask.

Notes and other records

Patient's notes, radiograph request forms and laboratory instruction card should be available.

Instruments and materials

- Mirror probe and tweezers – for general intra oral examination
- Ruler – to measure overjet and overbite
- Dividers – for tooth width measurement
- Intra oral mirror – for intra oral photographs
- Mixing bowl, room temperature water, mixing spatula, alginate and sealable bag – for impression taking
- Wax – for a wax bite
- Impression trays and a fixative
- Kidney dish – in case of vomiting
- Safety glasses for the patient, DN and orthodontist
- Gloves for the DN and orthodontist
- Protective bib for the patient
- Rinse water for the patient
- Hand mirror for the patient.

Chairside support

Duties may include:

- passing of instruments
- mixing alginate and loading the trays
- heating up the wax for the wax bite
- holding the intra oral mirror for photographs.

After treatment

Duties may include:

- safe disposal of clinical waste and sharps
- preparing the instruments for sterilisation
- sterilising the instruments
- disinfecting the work surfaces
- disinfecting the alginate impressions and packing them ready for sending to the laboratory
- arranging the patient's next appointment
- processing the radiographs – ensuring the name and date on each radiograph are correct
- recording the photographic film frame numbers next to the patients' name
- preparing the clinical environment for the next patient.

Patient care

Patient care is paramount during each clinical session and the DN plays a vital role in ensuring the patient is comfortable, safe and informed of what may happen during treatment. The orthodontist may also ask the DN if they can give oral health education to the patient (if they are suitably qualified), and also to inform the patient on how to care for their orthodontic appliance.

Other aspects of patient care would include:

- making sure the patient is wearing protective glasses and a bib during treatment;
- providing the patient with a mouthwash and tissue after impression taking;
- monitoring the patient throughout treatment.

Second visit – removable appliances

Preparation of clinical area

As with the first visit.

Notes and other records

Patient's notes, radiographs, photographs and models should be available.

Instruments and materials

○ Mirror, probe, tweezers, ruler and dividers

○ The removable appliance – may come with a key to turn the expansion screw

○ Rigid plastic container –to keep the appliance in when out of the mouth

○ Adams pliers – for adjusting the Adams cribs (Figure 10.23)

○ Spring forming pliers – for adjusting the springs (Figure 10.24)

○ Mauns wire cutters (Figure 10.25)

○ Acrylic trimming bur and straight handpiece – for adjusting the acrylic baseplate

○ Chinagraph pencil – for marking where adjustments may need to be made

○ Safety glasses for the patient, DN and orthodontist

○ Gloves for the DN and orthodontist

○ Protective bib for the patient

○ Hand mirror for the patient

○ Care of appliance instruction sheet for the patient.

Chairside support

Duties may include the passing of instruments.

After treatment

Duties may include:

○ safe disposal of clinical waste and sharps

○ preparing the instruments for sterilisation

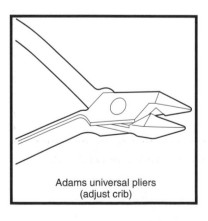

Figure 10.23: Adams universal pliers.

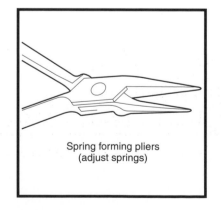

Figure 10.24: Spring forming pliers.

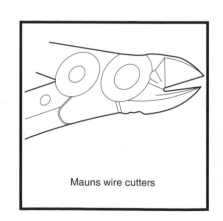

Figure 10.25: Mauns wire cutters.

○ sterilising the instruments

○ disinfecting the work surfaces

○ arranging the patient's next appointment

○ preparing the clinical environment for the next patient.

Patient care

Aspects of patient care may include:

○ making sure the patient is wearing protective glasses and a bib during treatment

○ monitoring the patient throughout treatment

○ showing the patient how to remove and replace the removable appliance

○ oral hygiene instruction

○ advice on turning the expansion screw (if applicable)

○ providing the patient with a leaflet on care of the appliance.

Second visit – fixed appliances

This visit, which is normally arranged about one week before the bands are to be fitted, involves placing separating elastics between the molar teeth to push them apart gently, creating space for the bands (Figure 10.26).

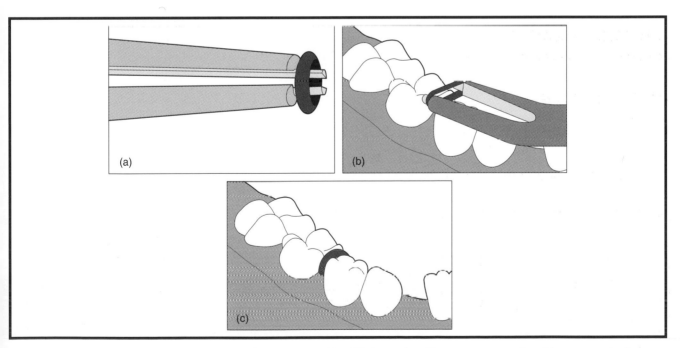

Figure 10.26: Placing separating elastics – (a) elastic on separating pliers; (b) elastic placed between contact points; (c) separator elastic in place.

Preparation of clinical area

As with the first visit.

Notes and other records

Patient's notes, radiographs, photographs and models should be available.

Instruments and materials

- ○ Mirror, straight probe, tweezers, ruler and dividers

- ○ Separating elastics – to be placed between the molars for about one week to push them apart ready for fitting the bands. Sometimes separating springs may be used instead

- ○ Separating pliers.

- ○ Water/air nozzle

- ○ Aspirating tips

- ○ Safety glasses for the patient, DN and orthodontist

- ○ Gloves for the DN and orthodontist

- ○ Protective bib for the patient

- ○ Hand mirror for the patient

- ○ Instruction sheet for the patient.

Chairside support

Duties may include:

- ○ passing of instruments

- ○ placing the separating elastics on the pliers

- ○ aspirating

- ○ gently blowing air onto the teeth to be separated.

After treatment

Duties as for the removable appliance visit.

Patient care

Aspects of patient care may include:

- ○ making sure the patient is wearing protective glasses and a bib during treatment

- ○ monitoring the patient throughout treatment

- ○ reassuring them whist the separating elastics are being placed between the teeth.

The separating elastics will cause the patient some discomfort as the teeth are being pushed apart. The patient should be made aware of this, and the orthodontist can recommend pain relief (whatever the patient may take for a headache). Care should be taken to check for drug interactions and history of any allergies.

Third visit – fixed appliances

Preparation of clinical area
As with the first visit.

Notes and other records
Patient's notes, radiographs, photographs and models should be available.

Instruments and materials (Figure 10.27)

- Mirror, straight probe (often a short ended one is used to make bracket placing easier), tweezers, ruler and dividers
- Arch-form card – to aid the orthodontist when bending the wire into an arch-form
- Brackets and bands – for cementing onto the teeth. For the straight wire system brackets are usually placed on a labelled sticky pad to ensure the correct brackets are placed on each tooth
- Archwire – normally a round nickel titanium wire for the early stages of treatment
- Howe pliers or Weingarts pliers – for holding on to the archwire (Figure 10.27a)
- Bracket holding pliers – for holding onto the brackets. Tweezers can be used instead
- Distal end cutters – for cutting the archwire. Designed especially for holding on to the wire when cut in the mouth to prevent trauma and inhalation (Figure 10.27b)
- Band seating instruments – band pusher, bite stick, oval amalgam plugger (Figure 10.27c)
- Bond removing pliers (Figure 10.27d)
- Lightwire pliers – for making bends in the archwire (Figure 10.27e)
- Mosquito artery forceps – normally small curved ones for passing elastic modules
- Ligature lockers – for the tying in of ligatures (Figures 10.27g)
- Ligature tuckers – for tucking the ends of wire ligatures safely under the bracket to prevent trauma (Figure 10.27h)
- Ligature cutters (Figure 10.27f)
- Contra angled handpiece and polishing cup
- Plastic cheek retractors – for maintaining a clear field of vision during bonding and banding (Figure 10.27i)
- Chinagraph pencil – for marking where bends need to be made in the archwire
- Acid etch liquid, composite material and curing light – for bonding brackets onto the teeth
- Glass ionomer cement – for cementing the bands to the molar teeth
- Non fluoride polish – for polishing the teeth prior to etching
- Water/air nozzle

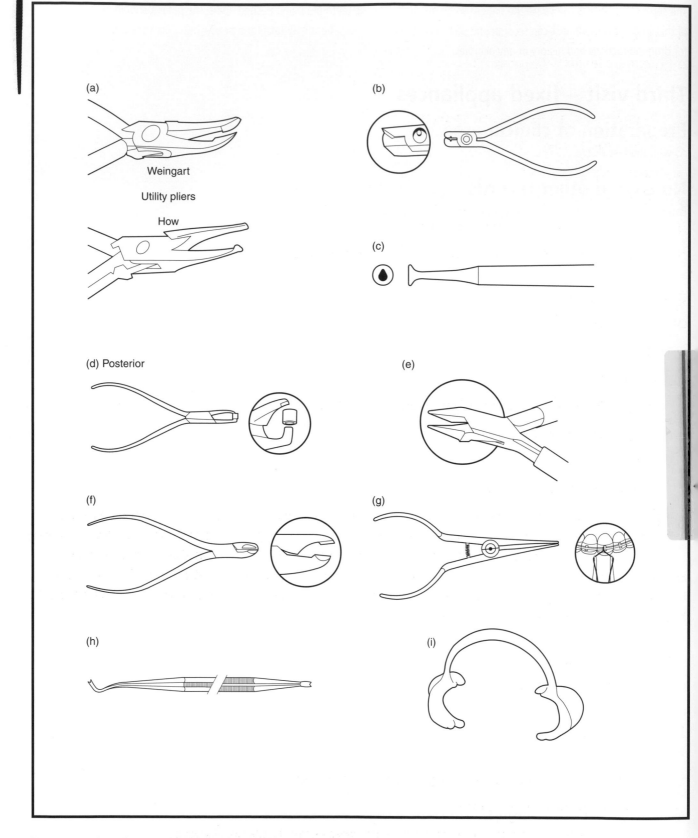

(a)

Weingart

Utility pliers

How

(b)

(c)

(d) Posterior

(e)

(f)

(g)

(h)

(i)

Figure 10.27: (a) Utility pliers (b) Distal end cutters (c) Band seater (d) Band removing pliers (e) Light wire pliers (f) Pin and ligature cutters (g) Ligature lockers (h) Ligature tucker (i) cheek retractors.

- Aspirating tips

- Mixing pads and spatulas

- Protective shield for light curing machine

- Cotton wool rolls

- Safety glasses for the patient, DN and orthodontist

- Gloves for the DN and orthodontist

- Protective bib for the patient

- Hand mirror for the patient

- Care of appliance instruction sheet for the patient

- Wax for the patient to place over any areas of the appliance that may be rubbing.

Chairside support

Duties may include:

- passing of instruments

- mixing materials

- placing bonding material on brackets and passing them to the orthodontist

- placing cement on bands and passing them to the orthodontist

- aspirating

- passing elastic modules and ligatures.

☞ Preparation of the teeth for bracket and band placing is an important part of this visit and it is essential that the DN and orthodontist work together effectively. It is vital that the etched and dried teeth do not get contaminated with saliva otherwise the bond between brackets and tooth may fail. Also a band cemented in a wet environment will run the risk of failure and become loose. Excellent aspiration, moisture control and ensuring the orthodontist has a clear field of vision will help maintain a high standard of bonding and banding during this visit. Other areas to check are that all the cementing and bonding materials are well within their sell-by-date and are mixed according to manufacturers' instructions.

After treatment

- Duties as for the removable appliance visit.

Patient care

Aspects of patient care may include:

- making sure the patient is wearing protective glasses and a bib during treatment

- monitoring the patient throughout treatment

- ensuring that the patient is protected from soft-tissue damage when etching, by effective aspiration

- showing the patient the appliance fitted in their mouth with a mirror before they leave the surgery

- giving oral hygiene instruction, diet advice and instructions on care of the appliance

- providing the patient with a leaflet on care of the appliance

- providing the patient with soft wax to place on any areas of the appliance that may cause irritation.

Further visits

Removable appliance

The appliance will probably be adjusted slightly at each visit and mid-treatment models and photographs may be taken. ☞ It is important that the patient's oral hygiene is monitored, and they are continually encouraged and motivated throughout treatment to care for their oral health and removable appliance to ensure a satisfactory outcome.

Fixed appliance

Further brackets or bands may be placed if a full bond-up was not carried out at the first visit. Wire ligatures may replace elastic modules and the patient may be asked to wear intra oral elastics towards the end of treatment to aid space closure. Wires would become progressively thicker and stronger and change from being round in cross section to rectangular. As with a removable appliance, it is essential that oral hygiene is monitored throughout treatment and the patient is given support and encouragement. Mid-treatment models, photographs and radiographs may also be taken. The patient may experience discomfort every time a thicker wire is placed, and they should be made aware of this.

Final treatment visit

Removable

The removable appliance may now become a retainer by holding the teeth in a certain position. The patient may have to wear the retainer full-time at first and then nights only, until eventually they can stop wearing it altogether. Some patients may have to continue with treatment by wearing a fixed appliance. Final study models, radiographs and photographs may be taken. The patient is given encouragement to continue with good oral hygiene and an appointment is made to check the retainer.

Fixed

During this visit the bands, brackets, bonding composite and cement will have to be removed. ☞ This can be a long, and in some cases, slightly uncomfortable visit for the patient, so the DN will play an important role in chairside assisting and patient care. Final study models, radiographs and photographs are normally taken at the end of the visit. Materials and instruments that need to be prepared for de-bonding and de-banding will include:

- De-bonding pliers – for removing the brackets

- De-banding pliers – for removing the bands

- Distal end cutters – for cutting the wire

- Weingart's or Howe's pliers – for holding on to the wire

- Composite removing bur – latch grip steel bur

- Mitchell's trimmer or equivalent for removing cement

○   Polishing cup and prophy paste – to polish teeth after cement has been removed

○   Contra angled handpiece

○   Air/water nozzle

○   Aspirator tips.

☞ The appliance must be removed carefully to avoid trauma to the soft and hard tissues. During removal of the composite bonding material with the bur and handpiece, the DN must gently blow air onto the tooth to prevent heat damaging the pulp. The patient will normally have to wear a retainer, which is either removable or bonded. If it is removable, an impression would have been taken at the last visit, and a retainer constructed in the laboratory by the technician. If it is to be a bonded retainer, then the DN will have prepared:

○   selection of thin or twist-flex wires – to act as the retainer

○   wire cutters – to cut the wire to the correct length

○   Weingarts or howe's pliers – to hold the wire

○   acid etch, composite and resin – for bonding the wire onto the teeth

○   light curing machine and protective shield

○   cotton wool rolls

○   aspirating tips.

The patient must be protected from the acid etch and the tooth must be absolutely dry and free from saliva contamination prior to bonding on the retainer. The retainer should stay in place for as long as possible, and will often need to be replaced if it becomes detached or loose. The most common area to fit a bonded retainer is lingual to the lower anterior teeth and the palatal aspect of the upper incisors.

Headgear

At the initial visit for the fitting of headgear the orthodontist will decide on the type of headgear best suited for the patient's treatment. This may include the following:

○   headstraps

○   neckstraps

○   Khlon face bows

○   J hooks

○   extra oral elastics.

The DN may also need to prepare:

○   Maun's wire cutters – to cut the facebow

○   straight handpiece and polishing stone – to smooth the cut portion of the facebow

○   Adams pliers – to bend the facebow

○   selection of extra oral elastics

○   tension gauge – to measure the force applied by the extraoral elastics.

Patient care

The patient may be worried about fitting and wearing the headgear, and they will need a lot of support and encouragement during this part of the treatment. The patient will be shown how to put the headgear on by the orthodontist, and then the DN may be asked to check that the patient, after a little practice, can place and remove the components safely before leaving the surgery. Headgear is often only worn at night and when the patient is at home. Most patients find headgear inconvenient to wear during the day or for school.

There are potential risks involving headgear especially injury to the face and eyes, so certain safety mechanisms are incorporated into the headgear. These include:

○ snap release straps

○ anti-recoil straps

○ plastic covering for the ends of wires.

The patient should be informed of the risks and advised never to 'play around' whilst wearing the headgear, or try to put it on anyone else. The patient is often given a record chart to fill in with the number of hours that the headgear is being worn. The more it is worn the quicker the treatment

SECTION 5: Health and safety implications during orthodontic treatment

It is important during orthodontic treatment that the DN is aware of all health and safety implications, and carries out effective infection control procedures. Orthodontic treatment involves a lot of wires and wire cutting, and special attention should be given to the protection of the patient and staff from sharps injuries. All wires that have been removed from the patient, and the clipped ends of wires, must be disposed of in the sharps bin.

A number of impressions will also be taken during orthodontic treatment, and the DN must be vigilant in effectively disinfecting the impressions before they are sent to the laboratory.

Information sheets should be made available for all members of clinical staff outlining health and safety and infection control procedures

SECTION 6: Oral health education, diet advice and care of orthodontic appliances Linked to DN24.1

Introduction

Prior to treatment the patient must attain a high level of oral health. Any underlying periodontal problems will compromise treatment and may cause long-term and irreversible damage to the support structures of the teeth. All carious lesions should ideally be investigated and treated if necessary, as it will be more difficult to carry out any restorative treatment if a fixed appliance is in place. Oral health education and diet advice should be carried out, before, during and after treatment.

Before treatment

Plaque scores

The orthodontist may request that the patient attain a certain plaque score before treatment can commence. In some environments, such as hospital or the community services, the hygienist may carry out this role. In some orthodontic practices, if the DN is suitably qualified, they may disclose the patient. It is important that the patient, (and parents if the patient is under sixteen), realise the importance of good oral hygiene before treatment begins. There are several different ways to record plaque scores and the orthodontist will decide on which method they wish to be used.

Method

The patient should be asked if they have any allergies to the dye used in the disclosing tablets, which is normally a vegetable dye called erythrocin. The patient must be protected with a waterproof bib as the dye can stain clothes, and Vaseline can be put on their lips to prevent them from staining. The patient is asked to carefully chew the disclosing tablet and than have one gentle rinse. The patient should look in the mirror and see the plaque-stained areas to give them an indication of where they are missing with their cleaning. A plaque score will be taken and recorded and the orthodontist informed when the patient's oral hygiene is good enough to start treatment.

Oral hygiene advice

The patient should be advised to use a small-headed toothbrush with medium textured bristles. When brushing they should use small circular movements with the bristles aimed at a 45° angle to the gingival margin if possible, (younger children may find a gentle scrub easier). For adolescents and older patients interdental brushes can be used for cleaning between the teeth, and adult patients can also be advised to use dental tape or floss. It is important to remember that, when using interdental cleaners, it is the sides of the teeth that are being cleaned rather than the space between them. The patient can also use disclosing tablets at home to monitor their oral hygiene technique. It is useful to provide the patient with an information leaflet outlining the advice that you have given them in the surgery.

Diet advice

It may be useful to carry out a diet analysis prior to giving diet advice, as it will provide a baseline to work from. The simplest and quickest form of diet analysis is the twenty-four hour one, which asks the patient to recall everything that they have consumed from the beginning of the previous day. By looking at this record with the patient, (and parent) you can pick out food and drink items that will contribute to enamel demineralisation, dental caries, dental erosion and cause damage to the orthodontic appliance when it is fitted. Foods and drinks containing non-milk extrinsic sugars should be kept to mealtimes only. Carbonated drinks if possible should be cut out altogether, or at the least reduced to mealtimes only. It may be useful to get the patient used to not having chewing gum or chewy sweets, such as toffees, before the appliance is fitted.

During treatment

Periodic plaque scores

Continue to carry out periodic plaque scores throughout treatment. Remember to ask the patient to bring in their oral hygiene aids for each visit.

Oral hygiene advice

If the patient is wearing a fixed appliance they will need to be shown how to brush around the brackets and under the wires using both their normal brush and interdental brush. Adults will find using dental floss and tape difficult, so an effective alternative is the use of superfloss, which will thread under the archwire. Patients who are wearing removable appliances should remove them for cleaning. If the patient does not keep up a high level of oral hygiene they may be at risk from long-term irreversible periodontal disease. The gingiva may also become so inflamed that it covers the bands and brackets making it difficult for the orthodontist to adjust the appliance and painful for the patient.

Check patient's oral hygiene aids

Always remind the patient to bring in their oral hygiene aids by having it printed on their appointment card. Check that the bristles of the brushes are not splayed, otherwise their effectiveness at removing plaque is reduced.

Daily fluoride mouthwash

At the start of treatment, the orthodontist may recommend the use of a daily 0.05% fluoride mouthwash, to help protect the teeth against acid attack and demineralisation.

Diet advice

The patient should be advised that they are to avoid consuming carbonated canned drinks, chewing gum and sticky sweets. All hard foods should be cut up into smaller pieces to avoid damage to the fixed appliance. It the patient consumes frequent amounts of sugary foods and drinks they are at risk from demineralisation of the enamel. White and brown spot lesions will permanently scar the teeth, which may only become obvious when the appliance is removed. Dental caries may also develop around the brackets and undermine them, resulting in treatment being delayed for restorative work to be carried out or treatment being discontinued altogether.

After treatment

Good oral hygiene, once established before and during orthodontic treatment, may continue after treatment and throughout life. Advice should be given on caring for retainers, especially cleaning around bonded retainers using superfloss or bottlebrushes.

Care of orthodontic appliances

It is important that the patient looks after and cares for their appliance, otherwise treatment will be compromised and delayed. The orthodontic surgery should be contacted as soon as possible when breakages occur, or if the appliance is lost. Some orthodontic practices will charge for replacement or repair of appliances if they are continually being lost or damaged. Breakages normally only occur to removable appliances if they are left out of the mouth other than for cleaning, and not placed in a protective container. Fixed appliances generally get damaged if the patient consumes inappropriate food such as chewing gum or bites into hard foods without chopping them up first. The action of chewing gum or biting into hard food will shear off the brackets from the tooth surface.

The DN, the patient and orthodontic treatment

The DN plays an important role during orthodontic treatment, not only in preparing the clinical environment and chairside assisting, but also in providing advice, relevant information and motivational support for the patient and their family. The DN also has to liaise with the orthodontic technician in the laboratory, ensuring impressions reach their destination and the appliances arrive back on time.

References

[1] *Essentials of Dental Caries*. Kidd, E.A.M. and Joyston-Bechal, S. (1997) 2nd Edition. Oxford.

[2] *An outline of periodontics*. Manson J.E (1983) 1st Edition. Wright.

[3] *A colour atlas of periodontology*. Waite I.M. and Strahan J.D. (1990) 2nd Edition. Wolfe.

[4] *Pathology of periodontal diseases*. Williams D.M., Hughes F.J., Odell E.W. and Farthing P.M. (1992). 1st Edition. Oxford Medical Publications.

[5] *Anatomy of oralfacial structures*. Brand and Isselhard (1994). 5th Edition. Mosby.

[6] *Contemporary Orthodontics*. Proffit W.R. (2000) 3rd Edition. Mosby.

[7] *Orthodontic notes*. Walther and Houston. (1994). 5th Edition. Wright.

11 MINOR ORAL SURGERY

Introduction

This chapter is linked to DN22.1, DN22.2, DN22.3 and DN22.4 of the NVQ Level 3 in Oral Health Care. Minor oral surgery can be anything from a straightforward extraction to a more complicated surgical extraction or procedure, both of which can be undertaken in the dental surgery. This chapter will identify:

❍ the reasons for extractions

❍ the equipment and instruments used in minor oral surgery

❍ surgical procedures

❍ the role of the dental nurse (DN).

Teeth may need extracting for the following reasons:

❍ treatment planning

❍ disease

❍ trauma.

Treatment planning

Sound teeth may require extracting for the following reasons:

❍ as part of orthodontic treatment if the dentition is crowded.

❍ the removal of extra, supplemental, supernumerary teeth or odontomes to enable other teeth to erupt or be moved into position.

❍ impacted lower third molars due to overcrowding or decrease in the size of both the maxilla and mandible.

❍ a badly positioned tooth to improve the design of a partial denture or bridge.

❍ the patient's general health. Clearances are sometimes advised before heart operations, and radiotherapy that involves the face or jaw.

Disease

❍ A tooth may be so carious that it cannot be saved or the rest of the patient's mouth may not warrant it.

❍ The pulp may be inflamed (pulpitis) giving pain, which may require extraction.

❍ Infection may spread from the pulp and lead to an alveolar abscess.

❍ Advanced periodontal disease.

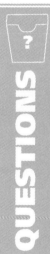

Trauma

○ A tooth that has fractured, loosened or been displaced.

○ A tooth involved in a fracture of the alveolus or jaw.

Forceps, elevators and chisels are the instruments used to extract teeth.

Forceps

A forcep consists of a handle, which is serrated to give a firm grip, joint and blade. The lower forcep beaks are set at right angles to the handle. The upper forcep is an extension of the handle. The upper and lower permanent molar forceps have beaks that fit into the bifurcation of the roots.

> **QUESTIONS**
>
> **?**
>
> **Question 1**
>
> **a. Look in a dental catalogue and learn the name, shape and number of upper and lower forceps.**
>
> **b. Write a list of the forceps and elevators in your workplace and what they are used for.**
>
> _____
>
> _____
>
> _____
>
> _____

Elevators

An elevator consists of a handle, shank and blade and is used as a lever to loosen teeth and roots. The most common are:

○ Warwick James (straight, left and right)

○ Cryer's (left and right).

The Coupland chisel has a concave blade with a flat end and is used by sliding the chisel down the side of the tooth into the periodontal membrane, thereby cutting the attachment, which will loosen the tooth.

QUESTIONS

Question 2

a. Have you seen a Coupland chisel used to remove upper first permanent molars?

b. What forceps and elevators would be used to extract the following?

D	6xx	3	8	4	1	7	6
1	1	7			8	65	2

Extraction methods

In the majority of extractions the blades of the forceps are slid down the root, or roots, of the tooth within its periodontal membrane. The root is then grasped firmly and pushed up or down and side to side to loosen and eventually sever the tooth from the periodontal ligament. The commonest way of loosening teeth is by expansion of the bony socket. The tooth is rocked buccally and lingually or palatally. The most effective is to rock buccally, as the buccal plate of the alveolar bone is generally thinner and weaker. Teeth with single roots, such as upper central incisors may only need to be rotated. When the blades of the forceps are pushed down between the surface of the root and the periodontal membrane they act as wedges, forcing the root out of its socket.

Elevators may be used as levers with the adjacent bone and sometimes an adjacent tooth if it is to be extracted. It is sometimes necessary to cut through the bone surrounding the tooth or root with a bur before it can be removed. This is called a surgical extraction.

The role of the DN falls into four main categories:

Preparation – Patient Care – Procedure – Post-operative

Although patient care is listed second it covers all the points.

Preparation

○ It is important to check that the patient has followed any pre-operative instructions.

○ Inform the dentist if the patient has not followed some or all of the instructions.

○ It is essential that the consent form has been completed and signed by the patient, parent or guardian and the medical history updated if necessary.

○ The DN should have the patient's records available and the radiographs displayed on the X-ray viewer.

- The surgery must be clean and tidy.

- The DN should set out the required sterilised instruments/items on a tray/trolley covered by a clinical sheet, out of sight of the patient until ready for use.

- Once the patient is comfortably seated in the dental chair, their clothes should be protected by a bib.

- Aspiration must be at hand.

- If it is a surgical procedure, aseptic technique must be used.

- An examination tray with a mouth mirror, straight probe and a pair of tweezers should be ready for examining the patient's mouth prior to treatment.

Patient care

- All patients should be reassured by a friendly and confident dental team.

- The DN must monitor the patient at all times, particularly during treatment.

- An appropriate three-way conversation between the patient, dentist and DN during the treatment will put the patient at ease, even if they can't reply, only acknowledge!

- Following treatment, the DN should ensure that the patient is feeling all right, there is no material/blood etc. on the face and that they understand any post-operative instructions given.

- Another appointment may be necessary,

Procedure

The DN should give close support to the operator by:

- Retraction of the lip, tongue and cheek as required.

- Effective aspiration ensuring visibility of the area and patient comfort.

- Passing the instruments, swabs and other items as necessary.

- Placing any removed specimens in a labelled biopsy pot, completing a pathology request form for the dentist to check and sign, then send for analysis.

- Monitoring the patient, e.g. change in blood pressure, skin colour, anxiety or stress.

- Alert the dentist if there is cause for concern.

Post-operative

- To give clear, concise verbal instructions, followed by written instructions for the patient to take home.

- Sterilisation of the instruments and decontamination of the surgery.

- Preparation of the surgery for the next patient.

☞ Post-operative instructions following an extraction

Instructions	Reasons
Do not rinse your mouth for 12 hours	This will wash away the blood clot and cause a reactionary haemorrhage
Do not drink hot liquids or alcohol for the rest of the day	Hot liquids can burn the soft tissue and may dislodge the blood clot Alcohol will raise the blood pressure, which will disturb the clot and cause bleeding
Do not do any physical work or exercise for the rest of the day	This will raise the blood pressure and cause bleeding
Eat or drink on the other side of your mouth for the rest of the day	If you don't you may bite your lip or cheek or both while the area is still numb
Take your normal painkiller if necessary	
The following day rinse your mouth with a warm salty mouthwash using one teaspoon of salt in a tumbler of warm water. Do this three to four times a day for at least two days	This will encourage healing
Brush your teeth as normal, being careful to avoid the treated area	
If bleeding occurs sit down and bite on a folded tissue for 20 minutes	This should stop the bleeding
If bleeding still persists or you are worried following your treatment, contact the surgery. If the surgery is closed contact the emergency telephone numer on the appointment card or go to your doctor or accident and emergency department.	

Cross infection control

In order to prevent cross infection, it is important that you use aseptic technique. This is a method used to ensure that the patient does not get an infection from other organisms during the procedure. If an infection were to occur it would cause the patient pain, and delay the healing of the wound. This begins with hand washing.

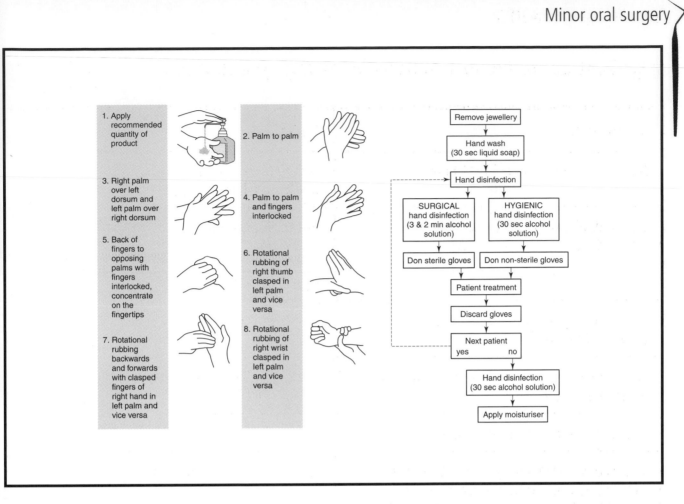

Figure 11.1: Handwashing technique.

Hygienic hand washing

Before hand washing, all cuts and abrasions must be covered by a waterproof plaster. Use a liquid soap and disposable paper towel. This hand washing technique is recommended for use between patients.

Scrubbing-up procedure

This procedure is only necessary when assisting with a sterile surgical procedure.

○ Wash hands thoroughly for half a minute.

○ Wash hands and forearms for two minutes.

○ Rinse so that the water drains off the elbows not the hands.

○ Dry hands first then forearms with a sterile towel.

○ Put on sterile gloves.

Gloves

The procedure for putting on gloves for a surgical procedure is shown below. It is personal preference whether the right or left glove is put on first.

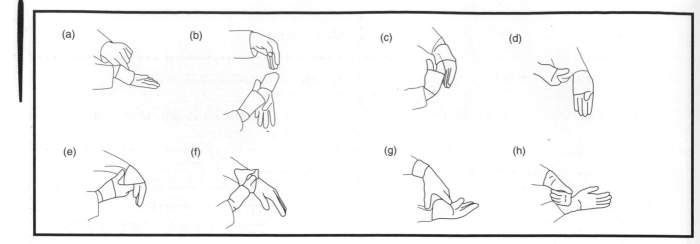

Figure 11.2: The correct technique for putting on gloves.

A Pull on the right glove by grasping the turned back cuff

B Pick up the left glove by inserting gloved fingers of the right hand under cuff

C Insert left hand

D Grasp outside of sleeve and fold tightly across the wrist. This prevents the cuff rolling, keep the left thumb across the palm of the hand.

E Hold sleeve with right thumb and insert right fingers under the left cuff

F Pull left cuff over gown at the wrist by spreading right fingers and rotating the left wrist

G and **H** Repeat as in diagram E and F with the opposite hand.

Once you have put on your gloves, you must not touch anything that has not been sterilised.

Differences between the maxillary and mandibular permanent molars

The lower third molar tooth is usually the last permanent tooth to erupt. Unlike the upper third molar, it is generally the most difficult molar to remove. The reasons for this are:

❍ the bone in the mandible is denser than in the maxilla

❍ more deeply impacted than the upper third molar

❍ it is larger and squarer than the upper third molar.

Maxillary	Mandibular
1. Triangular occlusal outline.	1. Square/oblong occlusal outline.
2. Crown often appears 'too big for its roots'.	2. Crown form similar to the lower sevens, but mostly smaller.
3. Largest cusp – mesiopalatal.	3. Four cusps.
4. Roots short, underdeveloped, convergent, often fused, curve distally. Usually 3 in number.	4. Two roots, short, underdeveloped, often fused, with a marked distal inclination.
5. Mesial contact only.	
6. Smallest maxillary molar.	

Impaction

Impaction is when one tooth prevents another from erupting into the arch correctly.

Causes of impaction

❍ Overcrowding of the dentition

❍ A decrease in size of the maxilla and mandible.

Forms of impaction

❍ Horizontal

❍ Vertical

❍ Mesio-angular

❍ Disto-angular.

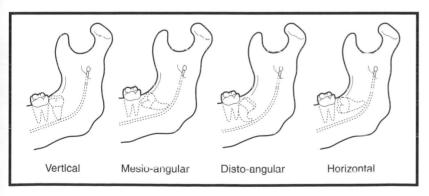

Figure 11.3: Impaction.

Problems of impaction

One of the main problems of impacted lower third molars is pericoronitis. This is caused when food debris/other becomes trapped under the flap of gingiva. If left, it will stagnate, become infected and cause the patient considerable trauma. This flap of gingiva can also become inflamed when the opposing tooth traumatises it during mastication. Usually it is suggested that the patient has the opposing tooth removed, as well as the removal of mandibular eights. If these teeth are left in they are likely to over-erupt into the arch, as there is no opposing tooth. It is also recognised that, if a general anaesthetic is indicated, then the upper eights should be removed at the same time to avoid a further general anaesthetic. If the maxillary third molar teeth are too highly placed and completely covered in bone they are left in place.

Consideration for choice of anaesthetic

❍ Proximity of third molars

❍ Difficulty of removal

❍ Patient's preference

❍ Any relevant medical history contra-indicating a local or general anaesthetic or conscious sedation.

Problems of removal

❍ Possibility of parathesia to the lower lip and tongue region. This is mainly due to bruising and swelling of the area involved and the close proximity of the inferior dental nerve and its canal.

❍ Possibility of fracture to the mandible during removal. This is more likely to occur in an older patient where the mandibular bone can be considerably thinner.

The patient should be warned of both of these problems, prior to the procedure.

Surgical removal of the lower third molar

❍ An incision is made in the mucosa using a number 15 scalpel blade and handle.

❍ A flap is raised with a periosteal elevator exposing the bone.

❍ The bone is removed with a surgical handpiece and surgical burs (sometimes a chisel and mallet is used).

The DN assists by:

❍ retracting the cheek and flap as required.

❍ irrigating the bur, tooth or root that is being drilled by irrigating with saline or sterile water.

❍ aspirating the saliva and blood thereby ensuring patient comfort, and visibility for the dentist.

Once the tooth is removed the flap is sutured back into position.

Question 4

a. Why may a partially erupted lower third molar tooth need extracting?

_____

b. Write in detail how a DN would assist the dentist during the surgical removal of an impacted lower third molar tooth under local anesthesia?

_____

_____

Question 5

List the instruments you use in your workplace for a surgical extraction.

_____

_____

_____

Other surgical procedures

Fraenectomy

This is the partial removal of the labial or lingual fraenum. A prominent fraenum may:

○ prevent or impede orthodontic treatment

○ prevent a good peripheral seal on a denture

○ prevent movements of the tongue.

Biopsy

The microscopic examination and diagnosis of a piece of tissue that has been surgically removed. In the oral cavity most biopsies are of the soft tissues. There are several ways to perform a biopsy, as follows:

○ Excision biopsy – the complete removal of the tissue plus some normal tissue.

○ Incisional biopsy – a portion of the tissue plus some normal tissue if the area is large.

○ Exfoliation biopsy – some of the tissue is scraped away.

○ Aspiration biopsy – if the tissue is filled with fluid it can be aspirated using a sterile needle and syringe.

○ Blood biopsy – blood may be taken using the same method as aspiration.

Apicectomy

The surgical removal of the apex of a root. This is only done as a last resort on a non-vital tooth:

○ Where root canal therapy would not be successful

○ Where root canal therapy has not been successful

○ Where the apical seal is inadequate

○ Fracture of the apical third of a root

○ Active infection during root canal therapy

○ Presence of a cyst

○ Curved root canal.

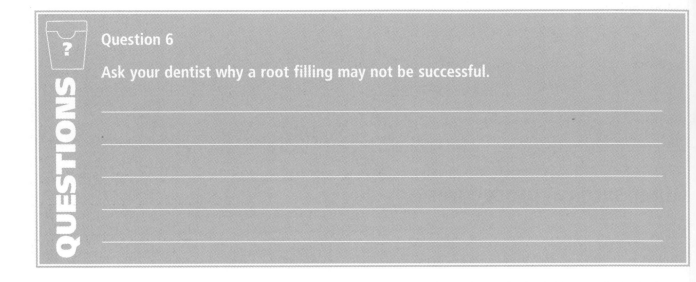

QUESTIONS

?

Question 6

Ask your dentist why a root filling may not be successful.

_____

_____

_____

_____

_____

Complications following minor oral surgery procedures

Dry socket	– Extremely painful inflammation following an extraction
Cause	– Usually infected and broken down blood clot
Treatment	– Irrigate the socket with warm normal saline
	– Pack with a suitable material to relieve pain
	– Advise regular warm salt mouthwashes and analgesics.
	– May require antibiotics.

Swelling	– May occur particularly following a difficult extraction
	– May last up to one week
	– The severity varies from patient to patient.

| Limited opening | – May follow the extraction of a lower third molar |
| | – This can last for a couple of days. |

Haemorrhage

Primary	– Immediately following the procedure
Reactionary	– Occurs a few hours after the procedure, due to the clot being disturbed
Secondary	– Occurs a few days after the procedure, due to infection of the wound
Treatment	– Reassure patient
	– Apply pressure on the area with pack
	– Give a local anaesthetic and suture area if necessary.

| Faint | – Refer to Medical Emergency Chapter |

12 PROSTHETICS
Linked to DN20.1, DN20.3

Introduction

This chapter is linked to DN20.1 and DN20.3 of the NVQ Level 3 in Oral Health Care.

Decay is not a modern disease. Seven out of 32 bronze age skulls found show some stages of tooth decay. Toothache has been the theme of many a medieval gargoyle. Look at the gargoyles depicted in your local churches. False teeth were found in Egyptian tombs; these consisted of natural teeth (from a dead person), which were bound together with gold wire or even string. The Babylonians in 5000BC believed, like the Egyptians, that toothache was a manifestation of the displeasure of the gods! Ancient Greeks made mouthwash out of calcium and pepper and had pliers fashioned specially for the extraction of teeth (although there was no anaesthetic!). Queen Elizabeth I suffered badly with her teeth and had many teeth removed, so she padded her mouth out with cotton gauze to give it shape. In more recent years, Winston Churchill had great problems with his dentures. They were connected posteriorly by springs, and no doubt it was the badly fitting dentures that added to his distinctive voice. Some of his dentures have been on display in the museum of a London dental hospital.

Thankfully, research and developments have moved on considerably and the materials and techniques now used provide the patient with a comfortable and well fitting prosthesis. With advances in crown and bridge work, removable prostheses (dentures) are not always necessary.

Prosthetics

The general definition of a prosthesis is an artificial replacement of a part of the body.

In dentistry this covers:

○ Crowns/bridges/implants/veneers/inlays – fixed prostheses.

○ Dentures/obturators – removable prostheses.

Removable prostheses

Complete dentures

These are used where all the teeth are missing (edentulous: without natural teeth).

Partial dentures

These are used where some or all of the teeth are present (dentate: having natural teeth).

Over dentures (also overlay and onlay)

These dentures restore function and appearance by covering the worn occlusal surface of the retained teeth as well as replacing missing teeth.

Immediate replacement dentures

These can be full or partial dentures. They are supplied when the patient needs to have anterior teeth extracted but does not want to go without teeth while the healing process takes place. As the bone resorption, which takes place following extractions, can affect the fit of dentures, any posterior teeth are removed and allowed to heal; impressions are then taken for the dentures and the anterior teeth are extracted at the same time as the denture is fitted. The patient will need to be aware that the denture may need to be relined after six /eight weeks due to the excessive bone resorption in the first eight weeks following extractions.

Obturators

These are devices made to cover a defect of the palate, due to:

○ congenital defects (e.g. cleft palate)

○ Surgical defects (e.g. removal of cysts or tumours in the maxilla).

Obturators can be complete or partial.

Preparation of the mouth prior to provision of dentures

Complete dentures

○ Removal of buried roots or teeth. Buried teeth that have no sign of erupting and are infection and symptom free may be left undisturbed.

○ Removal of bony sharp edges in the alveolar and also sharp mylohoid ridges.

○ Removal of denture granulomata – hyperplasia.

○ Infections should be treated as fungal disorders, such as stomatitis.

○ Any trauma present should be improved with tissue conditioners.

Partial dentures

○ Necessary fillings. Scaling and polishing.

○ Periodontal treatment and surgery where necessary.

○ Crowns, inlays etc.

○ Trimming down and correcting over erupted teeth.

Reasons for missing teeth

○ Periodontal disease (major cause of tooth loss)

○ Dental caries (dental education has seen a fall in dental caries in recent years)

○ Trauma (upper incisors are most at risk)

○ Planned extractions (planned extractions rarely result in the need for dentures, when the need occurs it is usually due to unsightly or malpositioned teeth)

○ Congenital absence (upper laterals are the most commonly missing teeth).

Other less common causes of tooth loss:

○ Anodontia (developmental absence of teeth)

○ Hypodontia (partial developmental absence of teeth)

○ Amelogenesis imperfecta (imperfect enamel formation)

○ Dentinogenesis imperfecta (imperfect dentine formation)

○ Stained teeth (tetracycline staining)

○ Resorption of teeth (roots of teeth close to cyst formation)

○ Cysts and neoplasm (bone loss incurred).

Consequences of partial tooth loss

○ Drifting or tilting of adjacent remaining teeth

○ Rotation of teeth

○ Over eruption of teeth

○ Loss of contact area

○ Formation of food traps following the above causes

○ Increased susceptibility to caries and periodontal disease

○ Occulsal disruption

○ Poor aesthetics

○ Localised alveolar bone loss

○ Increased likelihood of further tooth loss

○ Fibrous replacement of upper anterior ridge.

Consequences of complete tooth loss

○ Alveolar bone resorption

○ Anatomical suture exposed by alveolar resumption

○ Reduced masticatory efficiency

○ Faulty speech

○ Changes in appearance – prematurely aged

○ Psychological changes.

Purpose of partial or complete dentures

○ Aesthetics

○ Mastication

○ Speech

○ Training for future complete dentures (partial)

○ Health of oral cavity

○ General health.

Examination for consultation for removable prosthetics (dentures)

The patient's history should be taken, including:

○ personal details

○ reason for attendance (e.g. appearance/eating ability/ pain)

○ dental history (e.g. previous dentures)

○ medical history (e.g. diabetes)

○ social history (ability to attend/financial/NHS/private).

The extra oral examination is of special significance when considering prosthetics. The examination will cover the following:

○ General appearance

○ Bearing or manner

○ Appearance of present teeth both real and artificial

○ Clenching or grinding habits

○ Swelling or disproportion of face

○ Facial colour, sweating, facial tics

○ Skeletal shape

○ Temporomandibular joint function.

The intra oral examination will cover:

○ Condition of any remaining teeth

○ Periodontal condition

○ Occlusion

○ Possibility of any retained roots buried and visible.

Question 1

Why is it necessary to take into consideration the complete oral appearance when providing a partial removable prosthesis?

_____

_____

_____

_____

Medical conditions that directly affect the mouth need to be considered and may reflect on the type of prosthesis provided and its expected success. The list below is not exhaustive.

- Anaemia (soreness of tongue)
- Cerebro-vascularthrombosis (loss of movement, muscle tone and feeling)
- Arthritic disease (may affect TMJ in rare cases)
- Diabetes (susceptible to infection/increased bone resorption)
- Epilepsy (danger of fracturing acrylic dentures is very real)
- Parkinson's disease (loss of muscle co-ordination)
- Allergies (sensitivity to certain materials, e.g. metals)
- Cerebral vascular accident (stroke) (loss of muscle action).

Question 2

Complete a case study for a patient who has a medical condition that affects the provision of dentures.

_____

_____

_____

_____

Children and prosthetics

Rarely are children provided with removable prosthetics, due mainly to two reasons. Firstly, the constantly changing dentition until the full permanent dentition is complete, and secondly the acceptance by children of the impression and measurements required and also the actual life style of children need to be taken into consideration. However, in cases where through, genetic development, the dentition is absent or partially absent, the provision of removable prosthetics may be an option although even in these cases the growth and skeletal development of the child will involve the constant replacement of the prosthesis. Such procedures are often referred to a specialist paedodontist (dentist specialising in working with children).

Material from which removable prostheses are made

○ Acrylic

○ Metal – (a) chrome cobalt; (b) stainless steel; (c) gold.

Acrylic

Advantages

○ Lightweight

○ Inexpensive

○ Quicker laboratory stages than metal

○ Easier to repair and accommodate addition of further teeth if necessary

○ Can be relined in the case of immediate fitting.

Disadvantages

○ Needs to cover a greater area of tissues because they break easily and the stress needs to be spread

○ Greater coverage of tissues increases the risk of unhealthy tissues occurring

○ Not as retentive as metal

○ Not as comfortable as metal

○ Can affect speech more than metal

○ Can affect taste.

Metal

Disadvantages

○ Difficult to add any additional teeth

○ Expensive

○ Require more laboratory stages

○ Difficult to repair.

Advantages

○ Less movement within the mouth and therefore less damaging to remaining teeth and tissues

○ Stronger, less likely to break where single teeth are replaced

○ Last longer

○ Easier to keep clean. Less risk of fungal spores invading the material.

QUESTIONS

?

Question 3

Refer to your case study: What denture materials may be most suitable?

_____

_____

_____

_____

_____

Components and parts of a removable prosthesis (denture)

Identified below are the components for metal partial dentures, when the denture is constructed from acrylic.

Framework

The cast metal skeleton, which supplies the support for the saddle and retainers of a metal denture.

Major connector or bar

The section that joins the right to the left side of a denture.

Saddle

A metal mesh extension of the connector covered with acrylic. The saddle holds the artificial teeth.

Retainer or clasp

Provides additional support by circulating a remaining natural tooth.

Rests

A projection on or near a clasp, designed to control the seating of the prosthesis.

Artificial teeth

Constructed from either acrylic or porcelain.

Full prosthesis/denture

Identified below are the components needed for full prostheses/dentures.

Base

Fits over the alveolar ridge and surrounding gingival area. The base is usually constructed from acrylic. To provide additional support metal mesh is sometimes inserted within the acrylic.

Flange

Is the part of the base that extends over the attached mucosa from the margin of the teeth to the border of the denture.

Border

The circumferential margin of the denture.

Post dam or posterior palatal seal

Formed at the junction of tissues and the posterior border of the denture.

Artificial teeth

Either acrylic or porcelain.

Materials used in the construction of dental prosthesis

☞ The following materials are used across the range of dental prostheses. There are many brand names available in each category so it is wise to familiarise yourself with two or three of the different brands in each generic category.

Rigid impression materials

Impression compound

Composition: resins, plasticisers and fillers.

This is a thermoplastic material – when heated in hot (but not boiling) water above 55–60°C it becomes soft and will take up a new form. The softened form is placed into an edentulous tray and placed in the patient's mouth where it takes up the imprint and shape of the ridge. On cooling to the mouth temperature it hardens and can be removed, retaining an impression of the required element of the oral cavity. No chemical reaction is involved in the use of this material.

The retained surface detail on the impression is not as good as with many other materials. It is therefore used to, in effect, produce quick special trays in which a wash impression of zinc oxide and eugenol is generally taken.

Impression compound is rigid when cooled and is not suitable to record undercuts.

Impression plaster

Composition: calcium hemihydrate, potassium sulphate, starch, borax.

Uses: study models/first stage impression.

Mixed with water, measured accurately, working time is three to four minutes. The material is best used in a special tray as it records surface detail very accurately and the stability of the impression is good.

As the impression material is rigid once set it is not suitable for undercuts and dentate patients. It can be used as a wash into a compo impression special tray.

Zinc oxide and eugenol paste

Composition: Base paste – zinc oxide/olive oil/linseed oil/zinc acetate.

Reactor paste – eugenol and fillers such as kaolin and talc.

Equal amounts of base and reactor pastes are mixed thoroughly together on hard paper pad, to a uniform colour. The material readily adapts to the soft tissues and provides a detailed reproduction of soft tissues without causing displacement; it is rigid when set and is therefore not suitable for undercuts. Usage limited to edentulous mouths, within a special tray.

The zinc oxide and eugenol paste, although non-toxic, can cause a sensation of burning; the paste also clings to the skin around the mouth, and an application of petroleum jelly applied to the lips is advisable.

Zinc oxide and eugenol paste is commonly used to take reline impressions, where it is applied to the original denture. Either upper or lower, the denture is then replaced into the mouth until the paste has set. When used as relining impression it can be used for either partial or full dentures, the denture complete with the new impression detail is then sent to the laboratory for the new lining to be constructed.

QUESTIONS

Question 4

What reline paste do you use in your workplace?

_____

_____

_____

_____

_____

Alginate

Composition: based on alginic acid, which is derived from a marine plant (e.g. seaweed).

A fine powder form material mixed with the required amount of water. The problem of inhalation of fine dust particles has been overcome with many dust free brands on the market. The alginate powder can absorb moisture from the air very quickly; therefore the lid should be replaced on the container as soon as the required powder has been removed.

The mixing is done in a rubber bowl with a spatula, and the water temperature should be between 18 and 24°C (room temperature 21°C). The warmer the water, the faster the alginate will set. The alginate should be mixed pressing the mixture against the sides of the bowl to remove all air bubbles as these will affect the detail and strength of the impression. The alginate can be used in full or partial trays, either stock size or special trays. The setting time is approximately three minutes depending on the temperature of the mix. Alginate is suitable where small undercuts are present but has low tear strength.

Alginate impression must not be allowed to dry out, as this will distort the impression. The impression should be cast, if possible, within the hour.

QUESTIONS

Question 5

a. What alginate do you use in your workplace?

_____

_____

b. Have you ever read the instructions?

_____

_____

Elastomeric impression materials

Polysulphides

Base: polysulphide and inert filler such as titanium dioxide.

Activator: lead dioxide sulphur and dibutyl.

Equal lengths of both materials are measured on a pad and mixed to a uniform colour, taking care to exclude air bubbles. No putty version is used, so it must be placed in a special tray by itself.

QUESTIONS

Question 6

What brand do you use in your workplace?

_____

_____

_____

_____

Polyether

Base: polyether, a plasticiser such as glycoether and colloid silica filler.

Equal lengths of both materials are measured onto a pad and mixed to a uniform colour, taking care to exclude all air bubbles. Can be used in a special tray. The impression material is inclined to absorb water during storage and must be kept in a dry environment; the impression should never be placed in the same bag as an alginate impression.

Silicones

Base: silicone fluid and filler.

Activator paste: tetra-ethyl silicate.

Equal measures of the two materials are mixed on a pad to a uniform colour, taking care to exclude air bubbles. Silicones are available in putty form as well as light-bodied material. With elastomeric materials the environment conditions and temperature and humidity can affect the working time. However, typically the working time is 6 minutes and the setting time 13 minutes.

The elastic memory of these materials should ensure that when the impression is removed from the mouth any deformations caused through undercuts should totally and immediately recover. The impression is removed from the mouth with a sharp tug; this ensures that the material is strained for a short time only and that the elastic response will be obtained.

All elastomeric impression materials are hydrophobic. They don't like water – if the tooth surface is wet the impression material will not attach and fine detail will be lost.

Polyether impressions are stable providing they are not placed in a damp or wet environment, as they will absorb the moisture and the impression will expand. The new addition cured silicones are extremely stable once set. Condensation cured silicones will contract with time and should be prepared as soon as possible to prevent distortion.

?

QUESTIONS

Question 7

What impression materials do you use in your workplace and which group of materials do they belong to? How do you mix your materials? What care do you take to ensure that the material and the impression are of a high standard?

_____

_____

_____

_____

_____

_____

_____

Dental waxes

Dental waxes are mainly blends of natural and synthetic materials, bees' wax and paraffin being the main constituents, other substances in small amounts are also added such as oils, gum and colourings.

Commonly used waxes

○ Modelling wax: for the construction of dentures/recording relationship of upper and lower jaws 'the bite'.

○ Sheet casting wax: thin rolled sheets used in the casting of metallic dentures.

○ Inlay wax: small coloured sticks, used to record the inlay pattern, either directly in the tooth within the mouth or in models. The wax is hard and strong, easy to carve and to produce fine detail.

○ Sticky wax: white sticks – when warmed is adhesive to stick impression materials to trays, also used to hold fractured dentures together prior to repair, has various uses in this type of situation.

○ Soft wax: used mainly in orthodontic situations, a soft pliable wax. Small amounts used to cover wires, brackets etc. to protect soft tissues.

○ Carding wax: used to cover the edges of stock trays and also used to 'box in' impressions prior to casting up.

QUESTIONS

Question 8

What waxes are used in your workplace? Give examples of when and why you have seen these different waxes used.

_____

_____

_____

_____

Base plate

A thermoplastic material made mainly from shellac or a polystyrene material supplied in flat sheets. When moulded onto models forms the base of the bite registration.

Tissue conditioners

Used to improve inflamed tissues in the mouth, some are bactericidal. They act as a temporary reline material and do not require the use of a dental laboratory. Usually powder and liquid, comprising acrylic polymers and ethyl alcohol. The mixture is placed within the denture and positioned in the mouth to set.

Question 9

Write a case study where tissue conditioner has been needed.

_____

_____

_____

_____

_____

Acrylic

There are two types:

○ heat cured – used in the laboratory in the construction of dentures.

○ cold cured – used for the addition to dentures within the mouth.

Cold cure acrylic system can be used within the mouth to improve the peripheral seal.

Surgery stages of denture construction

The stages are:

1. Impressions

2. Special tray impressions

3. Bite registration

4. Try in

5. Fit.

Impression stage

Initial impressions are taken using either standard block trays (for partial impressions) or standard edentulous tray (for a complete denture) of a suitable size. The impression material often used is alginate. From these basic impressions a more exact fitting tray is made in the laboratory (special trays) in which a second impression is taken. The materials used in this impression technique are of the dentist's choice, but often an elastomeric material is used, which provides good flow and accuracy.

Set up

Equipment needed includes: mouthwash; hand-mirror; tissues; stock trays; tray adhesive; impression material; mixing bowls; water measure; spatula; gauze squares; plastic self-seal bag; laboratory form; disinfectant bath.

○ Selected trays should be fitted with a suitable handle, checked for size and sprayed with adhesive.

○ If compound material is to be used, sufficient cakes or sticks should be softened in a bowl of hot water and, when softened, inserted into a tray ready for the first stage impression.

○ Alginate material should be measured according to the manufacturer's recommendation, the tub containing the material should be shaken or inverted to aerate alginate particles – ensure that the lid is securely fastened! The measuring scoop should be used, the scoop should be levelled using the edge of the spatula, do not scrape against the side of the tub as this compresses the powder and will produce a dry mix.

○ Water should be at room temperature and measured according to manufacturer's instructions.

○ Mix well, smoothing mixture against side of bowl to remove air bubbles.

○ The mix should take approximately 30 seconds.

○ Load the tray ensuring there are no air bubbles.

○ Hand to operator.

○ On completion of impressions, assist the patient to clean their face.

○ Laboratory instructions should be completed and impressions labelled with the patient's details.

○ Impressions must be disinfected prior to sending to laboratory.

Occlusal registration

During the construction of prostheses the laboratory must have an accurate record of the patient's occlusion. The laboratory technician uses this information to articulate the casts so that the completed prosthesis will replicate normal jaw motions.

Face bow

This piece of equipment is used to record the relationship of the maxilla to the hinge axis of rotation of the mandible. The measurements recorded most frequently for complete prostheses are:

○ **Centric relation** (the jaws should be closed, relaxed and comfortable).

○ **Protrusion** (the mandible should be placed as far forward as possible from the centric position).

○ **Retrusion** (the mandible should be pulled back as far as possible from the centric position).

○ **Lateral excursion** (sliding the mandible to the left and right of the centric position).

The dentist will also record the following for all prostheses:

○ **Vertical dimensions** (the space occupied by the height of the teeth in normal occlusion).

○ **Occlusal relationship** (as occlusal registration above).

○ **Smile line** (the number of teeth that show when the patient smiles).

○ **Cuspid eminence** (the location of the cuspids).

Various measuring devices are used to obtain these measurements.

Bite stage

Equipment needed includes: wax rims; mouth rinse; tissues; Willis bite gauge; wax knife; Le Cron wax carver; hot air or bunsen burner; wax sheet shade guide; metal millimetre ruler; occlusal rim trimmer (or paint scraper); dividers; felt-tipped pen; face bow; Fox's occlusal bite plane; registration paste; orange solvent; spatula; plastic bag; laboratory form.

Special trays (if requested) are taken at this stage.

The procedure is:

○ Set out bite blocks (occlusal rims) on napkin with hot air/bunsen burner, wax knife and wax.

○ Set out the occlusal measurement devices, pen and shade guide.

○ Prepare registration paste if used.

○ If special trays are required, mix the operator's requested impression material – either alginate, elastomeric wash or zinc oxide paste.

○ Complete the laboratory form.

○ Assist patient to clean face.

○ Disinfect work.

QUESTIONS

?

Question 10

What measuring devices does your dentist use? Identify which measurements are obtained by each device.

_____

_____

_____

_____

Try in stage

Equipment needed includes: denture stage of teeth embedded into wax: large hand mirror: mouth rinse; tissues; articulating paper; dentatus articulator; Le Cron wax carver. If major adjustments are required you will also need: a hot air/bunsen burner; wax sheet; wax knife; dividers; Willis bite gauge.

The procedure is:

○ Set out try in stage of denture on napkin.

○ Set out articulating paper.

○ Dentures inserted and occlusion checked.

○ Articulating paper used to identify high spots.

○ Adjustments made to bite.

○ Evaluation made of fit and comfort of denture.

○ Evaluation made of function of denture.

○ Adjustments made where necessary.

○ Shade and mould of teeth confirmed as acceptable by patient.

○ Changes made noted on laboratory form.

○ Work disinfected and returned to laboratory.

Fit stage

Equipment needed includes: dentures in bowl of water; mouthrinse; hand mirror; straight handpiece and acrylic burs and rubber wheels; disclosing paste and brush; orange solvent; articulating paper; aftercare instructions; tissues; plastic bag for original dentures if present.

The procedure is:

○ Set out dentures in water on napkin with articulating paper.

○ Provide hand mirror.

○ Denture will be inserted and checked for functional ability and occlusion.

○ High spots checked with articulating paper and bite adjusted if required by using acrylic burs inserted into straight handpiece.

○ Patient given hand mirror to check appearance.

○ Patient shown how to insert and remove dentures.

○ Instructions given on care of dentures.

○ Further appointment may be given to check that all is well.

○ Original dentures (if any) wrapped and returned to patient.

QUESTIONS

Question 11

Identify the uses for the following instruments used in prosthetics.

a. Willis bite gauge

b. Articulating paper

c. Edentulous impression trays

d. Foxs bite plane

Question 12

Explain the following components of a partial denture

a. The framework

_____

b. The bar or connector

_____

c. The saddle

_____

d. Retainers

_____

e. Rests

_____

f. Artificial teeth

_____

Question 13

What are the advantages of a chrome cobalt denture?

_____

_____

Question 14

What are over dentures?

_____

_____

continued ▸▸

QUESTIONS

Question 15

Describe the role of the DN at each stage of the provision of an acrylic denture to an edentulous patient.

_____

_____

_____

Question 16

a. Why might an immediate replacement denture be provided?

_____

_____

b. What further prosthetic treatment may be required to the denture after fitting and why?

_____

_____

c. What oral hygiene instruction would the DN give to the patient after the immediate denture has been fitted?

_____

_____

d. What are the usual errors in mixing alginate impression materials and what is the result of those errors?

_____

_____

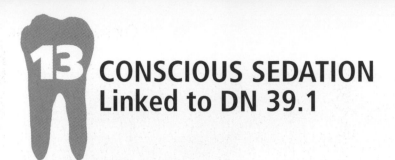

13 CONSCIOUS SEDATION
Linked to DN 39.1

Introduction

This chapter is linked to DN39.1 of the NVQ Level 3 in Oral Health Care.

The aim of this chapter is to provide an introduction to the use of conscious sedation for dental treatment. This subject is an area of speciality that is complimentary to dentistry and can be studied in more detail as a post-qualification course.

The dentist can administer conscious sedation to the patient, providing relevant training and updates are carried out. To satisfy the specific guidelines relating to the use of sedation in the dental environment, there must be a suitably trained person present throughout the session to assist the dentist. They must be able to clinically monitor the patient, have the necessary skills to be able to detect changes in the patient's condition and assist effectively in a medical emergency. A thorough knowledge of sedation techniques and the drugs used is essential. This person is legally referred to as the 'second appropriate person'. This is a role that can be fulfilled by the dental nurse (DN) who has attained a recognised level of proficiency in this field to meet the legal requirements. This is a rewarding extension of the DN's skills, which requires commitment and dedication. The General Dental Council guidelines to the use of sedation are comprehensive and legally binding for those practising this technique.

Definition of sedation

The General Dental Council defines sedation as:

A technique in which the use of a drug or drugs produces a state of depression of the central nervous system enabling treatment to be carried out, but during which communication can be maintained and the modification of the patient's state of mind is such that the patient will respond to command throughout the period of sedation. Techniques should carry a margin of safety wide enough to render the unintentional loss of consciousness unlikely.

Why use sedation?

○ To allay anxiety that the patient may anticipate or experience during dental treatment.

○ To reduce the stress associated with unpleasant or prolonged procedures. The effect of the sedation agent can alter the patient's perception of time and may produce an amnesic effect.

○ Can help reduce and control 'gagging reflex'. This reflex can make treatment difficult to administer for both the patient and the dental team.

○ Sedation can help stabilise blood pressure for those with a history of hypertension. Increased anxiety may increase the symptoms of the disorder, which can be alleviated by using this method.

○ To avoid the need to use a general anaesthetic. With the risk factor associated with general anaesthetics to consider it should be avoided where possible when providing routine dental treatment.

Question 1

If you use sedation in your workplace in which situations is it offered and why?

_____

_____

_____

_____

_____

Qualities of the sedation agent

When considering an 'ideal' sedative agent the following criteria should be considered:

○ Does the agent act rapidly to induce a sense of well-being for the patient?

○ Is it safe and easy to administer?

○ Does it suppress 'gagging' reflex, but not inhibit protective reflexes?

○ Will the sedative effect wear off rapidly following completion of dental treatment?

○ Does it provide a degree of amnesia and analgesia?

The sedation methods that can be employed following a positive response to the checklist are:

○ hypnosis – a highly specialised skill to create sedation without the use of a drug. Relies totally on suggestion

○ oral sedation

○ inhalation sedation also known as Relative analgesia

○ intravenous sedation.

In this chapter we are going to focus on the intravenous and inhalation methods. Inhalation sedation employs the use of low to moderate concentrations of nitrous oxide and oxygen administered from a specifically designed dental sedation machine via a nasal mask, together with semi-hypnotic reassurance and psychological support by the operator. The intravenous method requires an injection of a drug into a vein. There is a range of drugs available but drugs from the benzodiazepine group are commonly used. The drug sedates the patient as the only component of the technique.

☞ Local anaesthetic should be administered following sedation before dental treatment commences. Although the patient will feel more relaxed, the area for treatment will still require local analgesia to anaesthetise the appropriate nerve supply.

Assessment considerations

To provide the patient with an informed choice of options the dentist must consider the following points during assessment and discussion with the patient.

Find out the problem

Find out what worries the patient. Is it fear of the unknown? Or has something occurred in the past that has upset them? Discussion can be difficult if the patient is reluctant to revisit an episode that causes them distress. It is vital that a sensitive and reassuring environment is established between the dental team and the patient so that they can overcome this obstacle. Understanding the problem can ensure that the right option for the patient is offered, which will help reverse the negatives they associate with receiving dental treatment. It is possible that the patient may need more than one appointment in order to achieve this level of trust and openness with the team. It is important to listen to what the patient is saying, remember of all the skills we acquire during our development the only one we are not actively taught is listening. Often the patient may reveal pertinent points to you, in your capacity as the DN. This can happen during escort from the waiting room, while making an appointment or at any time. These points can be of great use to the dentist.

Dental history

This usually ties in with finding out the problem if the two are directly related. However, finding out what types of dental treatment have been carried out can provide an insight into the degree of dental experiences the patient is familiar with. They may not necessarily be unduly anxious or unco-operative but the dental procedure prescribed may be unpleasant or lengthy. In these instances it may be useful to offer sedation as an option.

Dental examination

A full examination is not always possible with a traumatised/phobic patient. In these cases an open consent can be obtained to cover treatment carried out during the planned treatment session.

Medical history

It is essential to obtain a comprehensive history following up any queries with general medical practitioners and hospital consultants if required.

Social factors

Finding out about the patient's domestic circumstances is helpful in determining which type of sedation is appropriate for them, e.g. intravenous sedation requires an adult escort to take the patient home and to be able to stay with the patient for the rest of the day.

Discussion

This should not be rushed. The patient should have the opportunity to discuss the options fully and will be required to sign a consent form for treatment under sedation. If they are still unsure they should have the opportunity to return to the surgery. It may be helpful for them to bring a family member or friend to the next appointment. Suggesting that they make a list of the questions they wish to ask is also beneficial. They should not sign the consent form under duress and written consent should be sought at the planning stage rather than at the sedation appointment, when they may be particularly anxious. On reflection it could be considered that the patient was not capable of making an informed decision, which would invalidate the consent to treatment if challenged at a later date. Every effort should be made to obtain a detailed consent form describing the treatment plan at this stage. The 'open' consent mentioned under the examination heading should only be considered when all attempts to examine the patient fully have failed.

☞ Written consent is essential.

Instructions

The patient must be given verbal and written instructions to accompany the sedation method chosen. When we are nervous it is difficult to recall all the facts discussed or the information can become muddled, which is why the written instructions should always be provided. It is vital that an adult escort is available to take the patient home following the appointment. This is mandatory for intravenous sedation.

The patient should be advised to eat a small meal before attending the surgery. It would be wise to check this with the patient when they arrive for the appointment as an empty tummy when you are feeling nervous can make you feel nauseous and prone to fainting. A glucose drink can be given prior to the session, which should help alleviate the symptoms.

Which method?

There are a number of methods.

Inhalation sedation

Advantages

- Non-invasive (useful method for those with needle phobia)
- Drug level easily altered or discontinued during treatment session
- Drug uptake and elimination via the respiratory system
- Minimal impairment of reflexes
- Recovery following discontinuation of drug within 15 minutes
- Amnesic effect (see disadvantages)
- Degree of analgesia
- Suitable for children. Generally used for children over 4 years of age as they need to be able to communicate fully and be at an age of reason to establish a rapport with the dental team
- Suitable for those with sickle cell trait.

Disadvantages

- Sedation dependent on psychological reassurance and effective operator technique
- Drug must be administered continuously during treatment
- Amnesia experienced by the patient is variable
- Not suitable for the over 25s. This is a subtle sedation technique that may not be persuasive enough for a resistant adult
- Nasal mask may interfere with site of treatment and offer poor access for the dentist
- Nitrous oxide pollution.

Contra indications

- Common cold or nasal obstruction. This causes mouth breathing, which would make this sedation method ineffectual.
- Pregnancy during the first trimester as a precautionary measure.

○ Mask phobia.

○ Traumatic procedures. e.g. impacted tooth.

○ Medical conditions affecting the central nervous system e.g. Multiple sclerosis. All sedative drugs alter the response of the brain regardless of the site of induction. The central nervous system delivers these messages for interpretation by the brain, so any damage or distortion of the central nervous system will inhibit the intended action of the drug.

○ Inability to communicate or interpret information and instruction by the patient.

○ Severe psychiatric disorders.

○ Cyanosis at rest caused by chronic respiratory or cardiac diseases. **Asthma is not a contra indication**. This type of sedation can actively ease symptoms by relaxing constriction.

Intravenous sedation

Advantages

○ The drug is administered remote from the oral cavity

○ Rapid onset of sedation

○ Co-operation from the patient less important. This technique does not require continuous psychological support during treatment, unlike inhalation sedation

○ Excellent amnesic properties

○ Single dose usually sufficient

○ Working time more predictable

○ No nitrous oxide pollution

○ Mouth breathing is not an issue

○ A benzodiazepine antagonist called flumazenil is available. This drug reverses the sedative effect created by the benzodiazepine. It must not be used as a method of recovering the patient to facilitate a speedy recovery and discharge from the surgery. It must only be administered in the event of a medical emergency involving the patient during the treatment session.

Disadvantages

○ Not suitable for those with needle phobia.

○ No analgesia.

○ Not suitable for children under 16 years of age. The drug has an unpredictable effect on younger children.

○ Unintentional overdose of the drug can cause respiratory depression.

○ Once administered the drug cannot be discontinued.

○ Laryngeal reflexes may be impaired or lost for a short time following induction.

○ There is the possibility of accidental intra arterial injection, which can cause damage to the arteries.

○ Occasionally the drug may cause a paradoxical effect causing undesirable and unpredictable behaviour, which may lead to increased symptoms of anxiety.

Contra indications

- Known allergy to benzodiazepines (BDZs)
- Alcohol or drug dependency
- Medical drug regimes that may interact adversely with introduction of BDZs into the body
- Children under 16 years of age
- Needle phobia
- Poor venous condition
- Pregnancy/breastfeeding
- Social factors, such as family responsibilities, carer needs or employment commitments
- No escort available. This is a mandatory treatment requirement, which will be checked before treatment session commences. No escort means no sedation.

Stages of the sedation process

Induction

In both types of sedation (inhalation and intravenous) the dose is given in timed increments. This is known as titration. The response of the patient and clinical signs are constantly monitored against the increments being administered. The amount of the sedative agent required to produce an effective relaxed state will vary for each individual. Signs of sedation can include some of the following: slower responses, although the patient is still able to carry out a command; slurring of speech, although they can communicate; their eyes may appear 'glassy' and 'dreamy'; they will generally look more relaxed and comfortable.

Maintenance

This phase needs to be monitored throughout the session, combining clinical observation with the use of mechanical methods. This would include the use of equipment such as a sphygmomanometer and pulse oximeter, which are compulsory items required during the use of intravenous sedation. For inhalation sedation the drug is administered constantly throughout the procedure. If there are moments when the patient becomes increasingly anxious the amount of nitrous oxide can be increased. With intravenous sedation the drug is already in the body and there is an estimated working time of 30–40 minutes from the onset of sedation, which is more predictable.

Recovery

The treatment has been completed and it is time to allow the patient to rest and recover. They may want to talk through their experience and it is important that all comments are positive and encouraging. These positive points will be the ones they take away with them. This may be the first time they have experienced a successful dental appointment, which will make continued dental visits less of an anticipated ordeal in the future. There are differences in the recovery time between inhalation and intravenous sedation. With the inhalation method the recovery time is rapid, usually within fifteen minutes. When treatment is complete the patient is given oxygen for five minutes. Nitrous oxide is eliminated rapidly from the body via the respiratory system. Speech and responses quickly return and they are able to walk in a straight line and hold their balance within this period of recovery. Intravenous sedation has a more profound effect on the patient and they should be allowed to recover in a designated recovery area where they can lie down for a while. Because of the nature of the drug used and the process of elimination from the body they will still feel slightly sedated for a few hours. This is why they **must** have an escort home and someone who can stay with them for the rest of the day. The patient should remain at the dental surgery for one hour following the last increment of the intravenous drug.

Post-operative instructions should be given verbally and in writing to both the patient and the escort. The instructions should include information relating to the dental procedure and instructions for the post sedation. If the patient has had IV sedation, the instructions will include: not driving; not operating machinery; not going to work; not signing legal documents.

QUESTIONS

Question 2

If sedation is used at your place of work what verbal and written instructions are given?

_____

_____

_____

_____

GLOSSARY

Abrasion: Wearing away of tooth tissue due to abrasive substances

Abutment: Tooth, crown or part of implant used to provide support for a fixed or removable prosthesis

Accelerator: Substance used in small quantities to increase chemical reaction

Activator: An agent making chemicals capable of reacting with others

Aesthetic: Appearance

Agar: Extract from seaweed, used for duplicating techniques in dental laboratories

Airway: Passage for air in and out of the lungs

Alginate: Common name given to irreversible hydrocolloid dental impression material

Allergy: Abnormal reaction to a substance that is normally harmless

Amalgam: Permanent restorative material containing a metal alloy, largely of silver, that is mixed with mercury

Amalgamator: Machine designed to mix the constituents of amalgam

Amelo-dentinal junction: Area where enamel and dentine meet

Amnesia: Partial or total loss of memory

Anaesthesia: Without feeling

Analgesia: Inability to feel pain

Anaphylactic shock: Severe reaction to a normally harmless substance can cause collapse and severe drop in blood pressure, can be fatal

Angina: Severe pain in the chest and left arm caused by inadequate blood supply to the cardiac muscle

Angle's classification: A classification of malocclusion, which is concerned mainly with the relationship of the teeth in an anteroposterior plane (front to back). It is mainly based on how the upper and lower first permanent molars occlude with each other

Anodontia: Developmental absence of some or all teeth

Anoxia: Lack of oxygen

Anterior: In front or before

Anticonvulsant: A drug used to reduce convulsions e.g. in epilepsy

Apex: Area at the top of the root

Arrhythmia: Any variation to the normal rhythm of the heart

Articulate: The relationship of the upper and lower dentition in normal movement

Articulator: Mechanical device to which models of upper and lower arches are attached and which records the position of the mandible in relation to the maxilla

Aseptic: Free from infection, sterile

Aseptic technique: A non-touch technique free from infection

Aspiration: Withdrawal of air, fluid, debris

Asthma: A condition causing difficulty in breathing; can be allergy, exertion, stress or infection

Attrition: Wearing away of tooth tissue due to tooth contact

Avulsed: Complete loss of tooth due to trauma

Backing: Metal component of a crown or denture designed for strength and to support the tooth-coloured facing

Bacteria: Micro-organisms often disease-causing

Bar: Metal segment connecting two parts of a denture together e.g. right & left posterior teeth in a partial lower denture

Baseplate: Temporary foundation on which a denture is built

Benzodiazepine: The descriptive name for a particular family of drugs

Bifurcation: Division where one structure divides into two

Bite: Registration of the occlusion by the use of wax or other material

BPE/CPITN probe: The basic periodontal examination probe, or the community, periodontal index of treatment needs probe. A probe used for periodontal screening purposes

Bracing: Portion of a partial denture designed to resist the action of lateral displacement

Bradycardia: A condition that slows the heart

Bridge: Fixed prosthesis replacing missing dentition

Buccal: Relating to the cheek

Bur: Rotary instrument used in a handpiece for cutting tooth tissue or bone

Calcific: Bridge or barrier following calcium hydroxide applications

Calcium hydroxide: A material that promotes secondary dentine

Callipers: Two-armed instrument used for measuring lengths used in assessing relation of maxilla to mandible in making of dentures

Cantilever: Bridge in which the pontic has only one retainer/abutment

Cardiac: Of the heart

Carotid artery: The main artery on each side of the neck, carries oxygen to the brain

Cast: Replication of a form e.g. crown, taken from an impression

Cast: Reproduction of impressions taken

Casting: Shape, usually metal, formed by forcing molten metal into a mould

Cementum: Bony tissue surrounding the root dentine

Ceramic: Items e.g. crowns made of porcelain

Chrome cobalt: Metallic element used to form alloys used in construction of some metal dentures

Chronic: Ongoing or recurrent

Coma: Complete unconsciousness

Composite: Tooth-coloured restorative material

Connector: Part of the denture that connects the saddle area or other components

Conscious: Awake

Contracted pupils: Small pinhead-sized pupils

Coronal: Relating to the crown

Coronary thrombosis: Blockage of one of the arteries in the heart caused by narrowing or a blockage

Crown: Part of the tooth that is above the gingival margin

Crown: Replacement of part or whole of the clinical crown, can be with porcelain, metal or acrylic

Cyanosis: Bluish appearance of the skin due to lack of oxygen

Deciduous: Exfoliation (natural loss) of primary tooth

Defibrillation: Use of controlled electrical shocks to restore the natural rhythm

Deionised: In this case relating to water. The removal of ions e.g. calcium

Demineralisation: Loss of minerals in tooth tissue

Dental caries: Decay and destruction of enamel, dentine and cementum

Dentate: Having natural teeth

Dentine: Organic calcified tissue forming bulk of the tooth, found beneath the enamel and cementum and covering the pulp

Denture: Removable artificial substitute for missing teeth

Diagnosis: Identification of disease using sign and symptoms

Diastemata: Plural of diastema, which is an abnormal space between two adjacent teeth

Dilated pupils: Wide-open large pupils

Dirty nurse: Someone who is able to get items for the aseptic nurse, without contamination

Displaced: Malposition of tooth

Distilled: Treatment of water for purification

Edentate: Having no natural teeth

Edentulous: Toothless

Elastomer: Impression materials with elastic-like properties

Electrosurgery: Burning away and repairing tissue using a low voltage (cauterisation)

Emphysema: Abnormal presence of air in the tissues or cavities of the body. Mainly related to lung disease

Enamel: Hard outer covering of the anatomical crown of the tooth

Endocarditis: Inflammation of the lining of the heart

Endodontics: Treatment of the pulp and root canal

Epilepsy: Disorder of the nervous system; can cause convulsion

Erosion: Wearing away of tooth tissue due to chemical substances

Etchant: Acidic substance used for the treatment of enamel and dentine for filling retention purposes

Eugenol: The essential oil of oil of cloves, various uses in dentistry including impression paste

Exfoliation: See *deciduous*

Exposure: Uncovering

Extracoronal: Outside the coronal part of the tooth

Face bow: Used in prosthetics to record the relationships of the maxilla to the hinge axis of rotation of the mandible

Facing: Veneer applied to the surface of a restoration or directly to the tooth to improve the appearance

Faint: Loss of consciousness for a short time. also called 'syncope'

Fibrils: Small fibres

Fibroblast: Cells that form fibres

Filling: Material placed in a cavity for temporary or permanent restoration

Finishing: The smoothing and polishing of teeth and restorations

Fissures: Small grooves found in enamel

Fixed prosthesis: Permanently cemented restoration to replace missing tooth tissue

Flabby ridge: Tissue has replaced the bone of the ridge crest creating a flabby appearance

Flange: Projecting rim

Flange: Part of the denture that lies in a sulcus

Fluorisis: Mottled discolouration due to high concentration of fluoride

Fracture: Breakage

Framework: The skeletal metal part of a partial denture

Friction grip: Relating to the retention of the bur in a handpiece by friction

Gag: To retch without actually vomiting

Gagging reflex: An uncontrollable response to retch

General anaesthetic: A drug, or drugs, that induce and maintain a state of unconsciousness and loss of protective reflexes

Gingiva: Soft tissue surrounding the tooth

Gingivitis: A bacterial-induced disease that causes inflammation of the gingiva and is reversible by carrying out effective oral hygiene measures

Glass ionomer: Tooth-coloured restorative material that bonds to dentine

Greenstick: Specific type of impression material

Grind: To eliminate high spots

Handpieces: Instruments that rotate burs at various speeds

Hydrocolloid: Dental impression material containing water, which is viscous when used, then when set becomes a solid gel

Hydroxyapatite: Mineral compound that makes up enamel

Hypertension: Abnormally high blood pressure

Hyperventilation: High rate of breathing, can cause imbalance of carbon dioxide and result in unconsciousness

Hypodontia: Absence of teeth during the developmental stage

Hypotension: Low blood pressure

Hypoxia: Reduced oxygen in the blood

Implant: A tooth or tissue that has been re-implanted. Metal pin or blade inserted into the alveolar ridge onto which a prosthesis will be fixed

Impression: Indentation of mouth and teeth in a material forming a mould

Impression: Imprint, from which a model or casting is obtained

Incisor classification: A classification of malocclusion, which is concerned mainly with the relationship between the upper and lower incisors. It looks at the position of the lower incisor tip to the cingulum (middle third of the palatal surface) of the upper incisor

Increments: Regulated addition/increase

Inflammation: Reaction of vital body tissue to injury. Signs are redness, swelling, heat, pain and loss of function

Inhalation: Describes the access route of the sedative drug into the body, which is via the respiratory system

Inlay: Restoration of gold or porcelain, which is made by a casting process and fits precisely into the tooth cavity

Interprismatic: Substance that is found in between prisms

Intracoronal: Inside the crown

Intravenous: Access route for a drug via an injection into a vein

Keyes concept: A diagrammatical representation (four interlocking circles) of the multifactorial aspect of dental caries

Lactobacillus: Bacterium naturally occurring in the mouth

Latch-grip: Relating to the retention of a bur in a handpiece by a latch device

Lateral: To the side

Lathe: Machine for holding and turning materials, used to polish and shape dentures

Lesion: Area of diseased tissue

Light-curing: The setting of restorative materials using a 'blue halogen' light

Lingual: Adjacent to the tongue

Local anaesthetic: Numbing agent restricted to one area

Luting cement: Material of a creamy consistency used for cementation of cast restorations

Luting: Cement substance used to seal crowns, bridges, and inlays

Luxated: Displacement from a natural position

Lymph: Clear body fluid originating from the lymph glands

Major connector: Main bar between saddles of partial dentures

Malocclusion: An occlusion where there is a malrelationship between the opposing upper and lower arches involving the teeth, the jaws or both

Mandible: Name given to the lower jaw

Mandrel: Rotary metal shank used to secure polishing and abrasive discs to the handpiece

Maxilla: Name given to the upper jaw

Microleakage: Infiltration of dental caries into tiny spaces around restorations

Micro-organisms: Bacteria, spores, fungi and viruses found in the human mouth, throat and nasal areas

Mucosa: Layer of epithelium covering or lining the oral cavity

Nasal pharyngeal airway: An airway that is inserted into a nostril and helps to keep an effective open airway

Necrosis: Death of an area of tissue

Non-vital: Pulp is dead

Obturation: Filling of a space as in a root canal filling

Obturator: Device for closing an unnatural opening. For example, following surgery for oral cancer, or cleft palate

Occluding surface: The contact surface of natural or artificial teeth with the opposing jaw

Occlusion: Normally referring to the contact between the occlusal surfaces of opposing surfaces of the dental arches

Odontoblast:	Cells that form enamel	**Overhang:**	Excess of filling material projecting into the area of the gingiva	**Periodontium:**	The support structure of the teeth, namely the gingiva, alveolar, bone, periodontal ligament and cementum
Operator:	Individual carrying out clinical dental procedures e.g. dentist, dental hygienist and dental therapist	**Overjet:**	How far forward horizontally the upper incisors are from the lower incisors	**Periosteum:**	Tough fibrous membrane covering the surface of the bone
Oral airway:	An airway designed to be inserted in the mouth, which prevents the tongue from blocking the airway	**Oxygen:**	A colourless odourless gas necessary to maintain life. Can be stored under pressure and used to supplement ventilation	**PH:**	The measure of acidity or alkalinity
				Phobia:	A compelling fear or dread
Orthodontics:	That area of dentistry specialising in the study of growth and development of the teeth and facial skeleton, and the treatment of irregularities of the teeth and jaws	**Pacemaker:**	A battery/electrical driven artificial device inserted in or by the heart, it controls and maintains a normal heart rate	**Phobic:**	The descriptive term for those experiencing abnormal states of fear
				Pin:	Metal rod used for the retention of restorations
Orthognathic surgery:	Surgery that involves moving the mandible, maxilla or both, to correct severe malocclusion due to skeletal pattern discrepancy. It is normally carried out in conjunction with fixed appliance therapy, and also when the patient has finished growing, (normally after eighteen years of age)	**Palatal:**	Of the palate	**Pit:**	Small depression found in enamel
		Paradoxical:	Contradictory	**Plaque:**	A soft, non-calcified bacterial deposit (70 per cent bacteria), that accumulates on the surfaces of the teeth and other objects in the mouth, such as dentures, bridges and restorations
		Parathesia:	Abnormal sensation of numbness (pins and needles)		
		Periapical:	Around the apex of the tooth		
		Perioconitis:	Inflammation around the crown of the tooth		
Over denture:	Metal or acrylic denture designed to cover the occlusal or incisal surfaces of teeth. A sound tooth is often used as a stabiliser for a denture especially in the lower jaw	**Periodontal disease:**	A disease of the support structures of the teeth	**Plaster of paris:**	Calcium sulphate powder when mixed with water sets to a hard solid substance, used for impressions where there are no undercuts
		Periodontal ligament:	Layer of fibrous tissue surrounding the root of the tooth connecting the cementum to the alveolar bone	**Plastic:**	Dental materials that are soft while being inserted into the tooth
Overbite:	How far the upper incisors vertically overlap the lower incisors	**Periodontitis:**	A bacterial induced disease that breaks down the support structures of the teeth and can eventually lead to tooth loss. It is not reversible and can only really be stabilised	**Pontic:**	Part of the bridge that replaces the missing tooth or teeth
				Post:	Metal rod cemented into the root canal of a tooth as retention for a crown

Posterior: At the back or behind

Prion: Protein structure associated with CJD

Prism: Rod-like structure of enamel

Proclined: Teeth that are forward of adjacent teeth

Prognosis: Expected outcome

Prone: Lying face down

Prophylaxis: Treatment for the prevention of disease

Psychological: Relating to the mind

Pulp: Blood vessels and nerves in the root canal

Pulpal: Of the pulp

Pulp capping: Treatment of a pin point exposure of the pulp

Pulpectomy: Total removal of the pulp

Pulpitis: Inflammation of the pulp

Pulpotomy: Partial removal of the pulp

Pulse oximeter: An electrical device that monitors and displays the arterial oxygen saturation in the body and the pulse rate

Radicular: Name given to the pulp in root of the tooth

Radiograph: Picture using X-rays showing internal structures

Radiotherapy: Treatment of conditions e.g. cancer, using radiation

Recession: Gingiva shrinking away from the tooth

Remineralisation: Formation of minerals in tooth tissue

Resuci bag: Bag valve and mask used to artificially ventilate a casualty

Retainer: An attachment such as a clasp that helps to prevent the denture from dislodging; also a restoration cemented into an abutment tooth and used as the retention for a bridge

Retroclined: Teeth that are behind adjacent teeth

Ridge: The part of the alveolar bone that remains after teeth have been extracted

Root: Part of the tooth found below gingival level in the bone

Saddle: The part of the denture that rests on the alveolar ridge, it also carries the teeth of the denture

Saline: Solution of salt in water close to the body's natural levels

Saliva: Clear fluid, secreted by salivary glands, aids mastication and digestion

Scavenger/ scavenging: Specifically designed equipment that helps remove waste gases and purify the air

Sedation: A state of relaxation induced by the use of a drug

Sedative: A drug used to reduce pain and anxiety

Self-shearing: Part of an instrument designed to break in the tooth tissue. For example, retention pin

Sepsis: Presence of pathological toxins in the blood

Shock: A condition in which there is a sudden fall in blood pressure, if not treated can cause lack of oxygen to the tissues and can be fatal

Sign: Visual effects seen e.g. blueness of the skin called cyanosis

Sodium hypochlorite: A mix of clean cold water and household bleach

Soft liner: Soft polymeric material attached to the fitting surface of the denture, reducing trauma to underlying tissues

Sphygmoman- ometer: Electronic or manual meter that measures arterial blood pressure

Spill: Relating to amount of amalgam material in a capsule

Splint: Rigid appliance

Stenosis: Narrowing of part of a hollow structure

Stephan curve: A graphical representation of the change in plaque pH over time after a glucose rinse

Sterile: Having no micro-organisms

Stimuli: Reactions caused by substances or other means

Streptococci mutans: Bacteria naturally occurring in the mouth

Sub gingival calculus: Calculus that forms below the gingival margin. It can be found around any site in the oral cavity and is black in colour

Sublingual bar: Connector that joining mandibular partial denture

Substrate: Substance on which an enzyme acts

Supernumerary: An extra tooth in the dentition (in addition to the normal number)

Supine: Lying face upward

Supplemental: Supernumerary tooth of normal appearance

Supra ginigival calculus: Calculus that forms above the gingival margin, normally at sites where the saliva ducts enter the oral cavity. It is creamy white in colour

Swab: Small pack of gauze used to clean wound or stop bleeding

Symptom: Change in the patient that suggests existence of disease

Symptom: Feeling felt by a person

Tachycardia: Rapid heart beat

Tempero-mandibular joint (TMJ): Joint relating to the temple and mandible for opening, closing and chewing

Template: A pattern or mould

Thermoplastic: A substance that becomes soft on warming but then hardens on cooling

Thrombo: When prefixing a word means blood clot

Tissue conditioner: Soft lining used for prosthesis to improve the condition of the soft tissues lying beneath the prosthesis

Titration: Similar to increments whereby the sedative drug is increased in measured amounts

Toxin: Poisonous substance

Transfer zone: Area under the patient's chin used for the safe transfer of instruments between dentist and dental nurse

Trauma: Injury or wound

Trituration: Mixing of constituents to a homogenous consistency. For example, amalgam

Tubules: Small tubes found in dentine

Undercut: Area of tooth or cavity that provides retention

Undercut: Where the alveolar ridge has resorbed leaving an undercut below the main ridge, making the construction of dentures more difficult

Vascular: Relating to blood vessels

Vasoconstrictor: A drug that causes the blood vessels to constrict (get narrower)

Vasodilator: A drug that causes the blood vessels to dilate (get wider)

Veneer: Relating to a cast restoration that covers or partly covers a tooth

Vital: Pulp is alive

Vitality: Relating to the status of the tooth being alive or dead

Wax: Soft substance obtained from plants and insects but also synthetically produced. Many varieties in dentistry and prosthetics. Types used in prosthetics described within the section on materials

Xerostomia: Dryness of the mouth

X-rays: Invisible short waves of radiation that penetrate body structures. Used to form a radiograph

Zinc oxide/eugenol: A material used for linings and temporary dressings

INDEX

Index

Index